The Complete
Cat Health Manual

The Complete
Cat Health Manual

RACE FOSTER, DVM

MARTY SMITH, DVM

HOWELL
BOOK
HOUSE

NEW YORK

Howell Book House
A Simon & Schuster Macmillan Company
1633 Broadway
New York, NY 10019

MACMILLAN is a registered trademark of Macmillan, Inc.

ISBN: 0-87605-675-3
Library of Congress Cataloging-in-Publication data available upon request

Manufactured in the United States of America

10 9 8 7 6 5 4 3 2

Dedication

This book is dedicated with love to our wonderful families. To be successful at most ventures requires a group effort, and to be a good veterinarian is no different. We are fortunate that our families have always been there, have always supported us and, as families, have shaped our careers.

A very special thank you to wife Lynne and children Trenton, Tristan, Katie and Keaton Foster, and to wife Kathryn and children Amanda, Megan, Katrina, Jessica and Johannah Smith. All of you give true meaning to the term family.

Contents

ACKNOWLEDGMENTS *xv*

ABOUT THE AUTHORS *xvii*

INTRODUCTION *xix*

CHAPTER 1—THE FELINE REPRODUCTIVE SYSTEM *1*

- Introduction *1*
- The Female Heat Cycles..*2*
- Disorders of the Female Not Directly Associated with
  Pregnancy *5*
  - *Vaginitis* *5*
  - *Ovarian Cysts* *5*
  - *Pyometra* *6*
  - *Cystic Endometrial Hyperplasia* *8*
  - *Chronic Endometritis*...*8*
  - *Acute Metritis* *9*
  - *Mammary Cancer—Breast Cancer* *9*
- Disorders of the Female as a Result of Pregnancy,
  Birthing and Lactation *11*
  - *Ectopic Pregnancy* *11*
  - *Dystocia* *12*
  - *Uterine Inertia* *13*
  - *Uterine Prolapse*...*14*
  - *Retained Placentas (Fetal Membranes)*................................*14*
  - *Prolonged Uterine Hemorrhage Following Birth* *15*
  - *Mammary Hyperplasia* *16*
  - *Mastitis* *16*
  - *Eclampsia (Lactational Tetany or Milk Fever)*......................*18*

• Disorders of the Male Reproductive System *19*
   • *Paraphimosis (Due to Hair Ring)* *19*
   • *Orchitis* *19*
   • *Cryptorchidism* *20*

CHAPTER 2—THE MOUTH, TEETH, GUMS AND SALIVARY GLANDS   *21*

• Introduction *21*
   • *Retained Baby (Deciduous) Teeth* *23*
   • *Dental Caries* *25*
   • *Abscessed Tooth Roots* *26*
   • *Fractured Teeth* *27*
   • *Malocclusion of the Teeth* *28*
   • *Gingival Hyperplasia* *29*
   • *Gingivitis* *30*
   • *Glossitis* *32*
   • *Tonsillitis* *33*
   • *Cleft Palate* *33*
   • *Rodent Ulcer (Eosinophilic Granuloma Complex)* *34*
   • *Tumors of the Mouth* *34*
   • *PICA—Depraved Appetite* *34*
   • *Foreign Bodies of the Mouth* *35*
• Disorders of the Salivary Glands *37*
   • *Excessive Drooling—Ptyalism* *37*
   • *Sialocele (Ranula)* *38*

CHAPTER 3—THE DIGESTIVE ORGANS—LIVER, PANCREAS
AND GALLBLADDER   *41*

• Introduction *41*
• Disorders of the Liver *43*
   • *Fatty Liver Disease (Hepatic Lipidosis)* *44*
   • *Liver Tumors* *45*
   • *Hepatitis* *45*
• Disorders of the Gallbladder *46*
   • *Gall(bladder) Stones* *46*
   • *Gallbladder Rupture* *47*
• Disorders of the Pancreas *47*
   • *Pancreatitis* *47*
   • *Diabetes Mellitus* *48*

CHAPTER 4—THE DIGESTIVE TRACT   *49*

• Introduction *49*
• Disorders of the Esophagus *49*
   • *Congenital Megaesophagus* *49*

•*Normal Regurgitation* *51*
•*Foreign Bodies in the Esophagus* *52*
•Disorders of the Stomach *52*
•*Gastric Ulcers* *53*
•*Pyloric Stenosis* *55*
•*Foreign Bodies in the Stomach* *56*
•*Gastritis* *57*
•*Tumors of the Stomach* *58*
•Disorders of the Small Intestine *59*
•*Small Intestinal Infections—Infectious Enteritis* *59*
•*Hernias and Bowel Strangulations* *60*
•*Foreign Bodies in the Small Intestine* *62*
•*Parasitic Enteritis* *64*
•*Tumors of the Small Intestine* *65*
•Disorders of the Large Intestine *66*
•*Colitis* *66*
•*Constipation* *67*
•*Megacolon* *67*

CHAPTER 5—THE RESPIRATORY SYSTEM   *70*

•Introduction 70
•The Nose 71
•*Rhinitis* 72
•*Nasal Foreign Body* 73
•The Larynx 74
•*Laryngitis* 74
•The Trachea 76
•*Tracheal Collapse* 76
•*Tracheobronchitis* 77
•Lungs 79
•*Pneumonitis* 79
•*Pneumothorax* 80
•*Diaphragmatic Hernia* 81
•*Lung Cancer* 82
•*Feline Asthma (Bronchial Asthma)* 83

CHAPTER 6—THE HEART, VESSELS AND BLOOD
(THE CIRCULATORY SYSTEM)   *85*

•Introduction *85*
•*Cardiomyopathy* *86*
•*Vegetative Endocarditis* *88*
•*Arterial Thromboembolism (Saddle Thrombi)* *88*

•Heart and Vessel Birth Defects *90*
  •*Atrioventricular Valve Complex Malformation* *90*
  •*Patent Ductus Arteriosus (PDA)* *91*
  •*Ventricular Septal Defect (VSD)* *93*
  •*Aortic Stenosis* *94*
  •*Portal Caval Shunt* *94*

CHAPTER 7—HORMONE DISORDERS   *97*

•Introduction *97*
•Disorders of the Pancreas *98*
  •*Diabetes Mellitus ("Sugar" Diabetes)* *98*
•Disorders of the Adrenals *100*
  •*Cushing's Disease* *100*
  •*Addison's Disease* *101*
•Disorders of the Thyroid *102*
  •*Hyperthyroidism* *102*
  •*Primary Hyperparathyroidism* *103*
•Other Hormonal Disorders *104*
  •*Diabetes Insipidus* *104*
  •*Feline Endocrine Alopecia* *104*

CHAPTER 8—BONES, JOINTS, MUSCLES, LIGAMENTS AND TENDONS
(THE MUSCULOSKELETAL SYSTEM)   *107*

•Introduction *107*
•Disorders of the Bones and Joints *108*
  •*Polydactylism* *111*
  •*Open Fontanels* *111*
  •*Luxated Patellas* *111*
  •*Arthritis (Osteoarthritis)* *112*
  •*Fractures* *113*
  •*Tumors of the Bones* *115*
•Disorders of the Muscles, Ligaments and Tendons *115*
  •*Ruptured Cruciate Ligament (Knee Joint)* *115*
  •*Herniated Disc (Slipped or Ruptured Disc)* *116*

CHAPTER 9—THE NERVOUS SYSTEM   *119*

•Introduction *119*
  •*Head Trauma* *119*
  •*Tumors of the Brain and Spinal Cord* *121*
  •*Hydrocephaly* *122*
  •*Seizure Disorders (Epilepsy)* *123*

- *Infections of the Brain, the Spinal Cord and Related Structures* *125*
- *Motion Sickness* *126*
- *Cerebellar Hypoplasia* *126*

CHAPTER 10—THE EYE, EYELIDS AND SURROUNDING TISSUE *129*

- Introduction *129*
  - *Conjunctivitis* *133*
  - *Meibomian Gland Infections* *136*
  - *Entropion* *137*
  - *Ectropion* *138*
  - *Everted Third Eyelid* *139*
  - *Foreign Bodies Behind the Third Eyelid* *140*
  - *Prominent Nasal Folds* *141*
  - *Plugged Lacrimal Duct* *142*
  - *Epiphora—Tear Staining* *143*
  - *Retrobulbar Abscess* *144*
- Disorders of the Eyeball *145*
  - *Foreign Bodies in the Cornea* *145*
  - *Ulcers of the Cornea* *147*
- Corneal Ulcers Caused by Infections *147*
  - *Herpes Virus Infections* *147*
  - *Corneal Sequestration* *148*
  - *Trauma to the Cornea* *149*
  - *Hereditary Corneal Dystrophy* *150*
- Disorders of the Eye Chambers *150*
  - *Glaucoma* *151*
  - *Uveitis* *152*
- Disorders of the Iris *152*
  - *Iris Cysts* *152*
  - *Albinism* *153*
  - *Persistent Pupillary Membrane* *153*
- Disorders of the Retina *154*
  - *Detached Retina* *154*
  - *Taurine Deficiency* *155*
- Disorders of the Lens *155*
  - *Lens Luxation* *156*
  - *Cataracts* *157*
  - *Juvenile Cataracts* *157*
  - *Adult Cataracts* *157*
  - *Diabetic Cataracts* *157*
  - *Nuclear Sclerosis* *158*

CHAPTER 11—THE SKIN, HAIR AND NAILS *161*

• Introduction *161*
  • *Stud Tail (Feline Tail Gland Hyperplasia)* *162*
  • *Idiopathic Miliary Dermatitis*..............................*163*
  • *Ringworm* *164*
  • *Feline Endocrine Alopecia* *164*
  • *Neurodermatitis (Psychogenic Alopecia)* *164*
  • *Flea Hypersensitivity (Flea Bite Dermatitis or*
    Flea Allergy) *165*
  • *Solar Dermatitis*..*166*
  • *Skin Cancer* *166*
  • *Facial Alopecia* *167*
  • *Allergic Dermatitis* *168*
  • *Feline Acne* *169*
  • *Scabies*...*170*
  • *Cheyletiella* *170*
  • *Lice (Pediculosis)* *170*
  • *Cuterebra Fly Larva* *171*
  • *Fly Strike*...*171*
  • *Eosinophilic Granuloma Complex* *171*
  • *Abscesses*...*172*
  • *Frostbite* *173*
  • *Ingrown Nails* *174*

CHAPTER 12—DISORDERS OF THE EAR *175*

• Introduction *175*
  • *Auricular Hematoma* *177*
  • *Infections of the Outer Ear (Otitis Externa)*..........*178*
  • *Parasites of the Outer Ear (Ear Mites)* *179*
  • *Infections of the Middle Ear (Otitis Media)* *181*
  • *Foreign Bodies in the Ear Canal* *182*
  • *Hereditary Deafness*..*183*
  • *Deafness and Aging*...*183*

CHAPTER 13—THE URINARY SYSTEM *185*

• Introduction *185*
• Disorders of the Kidneys and Ureters.......................*185*
  • *Acute Renal Disease*...*186*
  • *Chronic Renal Disease*.......................................*187*
  • *Inherited Polycystic Kidneys* *188*
  • *Kidney Cancer*...*189*

• Disorders of the Bladder and Urethra.................................... *190*
  • *Cystitis—Infection of the Bladder*............................ *190*
  • *Urethritis*.. *191*
  • *Urinary Caliculi (Urinary Stones or Urolithiasis)*............... *192*
  • *Feline Urological Syndrome (FUS)* *194*

CHAPTER 14—THE LYMPHATIC SYSTEM   *197*

• Introduction.. *197*
  • *Lymphosarcoma (Lymphoma)* *197*

CHAPTER 15—COMMON FELINE PARASITES   *200*

• Introduction *200*
• Parasites of the Skin and Ears................................... *200*
  • *Fleas* *200*
  • *Feline Scabies (Sarcoptic Mange)*........................... *204*
  • *Cheyletiellosis—Walking Dandruff* *206*
  • *Ear Mites (Otodectes Cynotis)*........................... *208*
  • *Ticks* *210*
  • *Lice (Pediculosis)* *213*
  • *Cuterebra Fly*.. *215*
  • *Fly Strike*... *215*
• Parasites of the Heart and Lungs..............................*216*
  • *Lungworms*.. *216*
  • *Feline Heartworm Disease* *217*
• Parasites of the Intestinal Tract................................*217*
  • *Ascariasis (Roundworms)*................................ *217*
  • *Tapeworms* *219*
  • *Hookworms*... *221*
  • *Coccidiosis (Coccidia)* *222*
  • *Giardia*.. *224*
  • *Toxoplasmosis*...................................... *225*

CHAPTER 16—INFECTIOUS FELINE DISEASES   *227*

• Introduction... *227*
  • *Feline Panleukopenia Virus (Feline Distemper)* *228*
  • *Feline Rhinotracheitis Virus* *229*
  • *Feline Calicivirus*..................................... *231*
  • *Feline Pneumonitis (Parrot Fever, Psittacosis)* *232*
  • *Rabies* *233*
  • *Lyme Disease (Borreliosis)* *234*
  • *Feline Infectious Peritonitis (FIP)*......................... *235*

•*Feline Leukemia Virus (FeLV)* *238*
•*Feline Immunodeficiency Virus (Feline AIDS or FIV)*...........*241*
•*Ringworm*...*243*
•*Feline Infectious Anemia (Haemobartonellosis, FIA)* *245*
•*Fading Kitten Syndrome*...*246*

APPENDIX A—Normal Physiological Data for the Feline   *251*

      Role of Ash in the Diet   *251*

APPENDIX B—Feline Medications, Uses and Common Dosages   *253*

GLOSSARY   *255*

INDEX   *259*

Acknowledgments

No book is complete without giving a special thank you to all those involved in preparing the text. The employees of Drs. Foster & Smith, Inc., all play important roles. They communicate on a daily basis with dog and cat owners all over the world. It is through these conversations that ideas for a book are born. It is in these discussions that the concerns and desires of pet owners become clear so that they can be addressed in a book such as this. Tanya Frisque provided all of the typing and data input necessary in assembling this book. Candi Besaw, Mary Kinnunen and SueEllen Hopp helped proofread the copy for accuracy and ease of understanding. Patricia Dinda, our illustrator, provided all of the accurate drawings found throughout. Marcy Zingler of Howell Book House provided important editorial guidance. A special thank you to these six individuals.

Lastly, we are forever grateful to feline fanciers throughout the world who have supported Drs. Foster & Smith, Inc. We hope that by producing this book we have given a little back, or in some small way helped. By reading this book, your pets may live healthier and happier lives and give even more meaning to the term "Veterinary Profession," which we so proudly represent.

About the Authors

Dr. Race Foster is a practicing veterinarian with a special interest in feline and canine medicine and surgery. He has practiced in northern Wisconsin since receiving his DVM from Michigan State University. In 1983 he was presented with the 1983 Feline Medicine and Surgery Award by MSU for academic achievements in feline medicine. In addition to veterinary practice, he is co-owner of Drs. Foster & Smith, Inc., known throughout the world.

Dr. Foster is a member of the Michigan and Wisconsin Veterinary Medical Associations and resides in Rhinelander, Wisconsin with his wife and four children. Race Foster and his family all share a unique love for pets and have committed their lives to pet care. In his free time Dr. Foster writes veterinary articles and books and of course enjoys being with animals. He has a unique interest in consulting and working with professional dog and cat breeders, especially in the area of preventative animal health, and is a consultant on pet health nationwide.

Dr. Marty Smith's interests in veterinary medicine have included canine and feline medicine and surgery along with many hours devoted to wildlife treatment and rehabilitation. He received his DVM at Iowa State University and is a member of the Wisconsin Veterinary Medical Association. Dr. Smith has always played an active role in education. Currently he is an elected member of the local board of education.

Dr. Smith, his wife and their five daughters enjoy a wide range of outdoor activities including camping, hiking, boating, wildlife photography and skiing. Today he is co-owner of Drs. Foster & Smith, Inc. He divides his time between his practice, family, writing and consulting with organizations, breeders and other writers across the United States. Dr. Smith has authored hundreds of articles on various topics dealing with the health care of cats and dogs.

Introduction

It has long been stated that a cat possesses nine lives. As veterinarians who have participated in feline health care for over thirty years, we are convinced that this statement is correct with only minor modification. A cat truly has nine lives, but only one is of the body; the other eight are in the heart. The heart of a cat consists of love, determination, intelligence, inquisitiveness, desire, uniqueness, enchantment and independence. These eight factors simply add up to "a will to live." The ninth and final life is that of the body, a unit comprised of complicated interactions between cells, tissues and organs, all functioning in unison to create the physical element of life. It is this life that we as veterinarians try to maintain. The other eight are beyond our control. It is also this ninth and final life and its preservation to which this book is dedicated.

To live with cats and protect their health, one must understand the body, how it functions and what can go wrong. *It is the owner, not the veterinarian, that provides the best cat health care.* The veterinarian merely provides directional help; however, it is the owner who must ultimately recognize and comprehend that there is a problem and provide love and support until health is restored.

The goal of this book is to provide information about the most common ailments affecting the feline. This book is not all inclusive; it wasn't meant to be. The disorders discussed here were limited with intent to provide the best description of those ailments commonly encountered. It is assembled in an easy to understand format, an attribute we apply to our daily practice as well.

This book, being filled with factual and medical terminology, is not necessarily fun to read. That was not its purpose. It should, however, be included in the library of every responsible feline enthusiast, to be available when the need arises. It will provide answers to questions such as: What is ailing my cat? How serious is it? Why is it happening? What can be done? What can be expected? Much of this information is available elsewhere. However, it is not easy to understand. In the course of daily practice, a veterinarian is not always able to explain in detail. This book will help solve that. It is an extension of our veterinary practice to your home.

We hope that this book exemplifies our love of cats and provides you with an appreciation of their uniqueness. Cats do not appear complex, but they are; likewise, so are their diseases. Hopefully this book will help unravel this complexity and bring a simplification and understanding to their health care.

Please let this book help guide you through your cat's ninth life as long as life remains. By doing so, together we will have helped keep our beloved feline friends healthy and happy. In accomplishing that, our dreams as veterinarians will have been realized.

The Complete
Cat Health Manual

The Feline Reproductive System

The reproductive system is comprised of organs and glandular tissue, which function to produce offspring. The **female reproductive system** consists of two ovaries, two oviducts, a uterus, a cervix and a vagina (see figure 1-1).

A cat's **ovaries** are about the size of a pencil eraser and are comprised of glandular tissue and immature eggs. The ovarian tissue also produces hormones such as *estrogens* and *progesterones*. These female hormones regulate heat cycles and ovulation and control the uterine function throughout pregnancy. Eggs from the two ovaries are released into tubular structures called the **oviducts.** It is within the oviducts that, following a mating, sperm unite with the eggs to fertilize them.

From the oviducts the eggs pass into a large tubular structure called the **uterus.** Like the ovaries and oviducts, there are two uterine horns that unite into one uterine body. The uterus is "Y" shaped. The placentas attach the developing embryos to the uterine wall and transfer nourishment from the mother to the embryos. They also provide protection for the embryos. The embryos develop into mature fetuses within the uterus and remain there until born. At birth, the fetuses detach from the uterine wall and pass through the **cervix,** a valve-like structure that protects the uterus from germs such as bacteria. Once the fetus passes through the cervix, it enters the **vagina** and is finally passed to the outside world. The vagina also serves as an opening for the elimination of urine from the bladder, and it produces chemical substances known as **pheromones.** *Pheromones* are the potent chemicals that attract male cats to the female when she is in heat.

In the **male** or tomcat the important structures of the **reproductive system** are the two testicles, the vas deferens, the prostate gland and the penis (see figure 1-2).

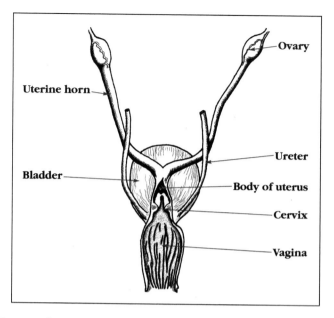

1-1　Female reproductive system

In contrast to dogs, male cats are born with their testicles already located in the scrotum; they do not descend later. The **testicles** have two important functions: they produce sperm and they secrete the hormone testosterone. Upon ejaculation, sperm leaves the testicles via the **vas deferens** and is transported to the prostate gland. The **prostate gland** adds fluid to the sperm to provide nourishment and aid in their transport through the penis and into the vagina and uterus. The sperm and prostatic fluids form a mixture called **semen.** Semen passes through the **urethra** and finally exits through the **penis.**

The cat's penis has some unique features. As a male cat reaches sexual maturity, usually around seven months of age, small barb-like structures or spines develop around the penile shaft. It is thought that during intercourse these spines stimulate the vaginal wall and cause a production of hormones in the female, which aid in ovulation. The penis of the cat is rather small when compared to other mammals and is protected in a hair-covered sheath or prepuce. Because of its small size and protective sheath it is not easily exposed for examination.

THE FEMALE HEAT CYCLES

Unlike dogs and humans, female cats do not cycle at regular intervals throughout the year. Cats tend to come in heat in relation to the season

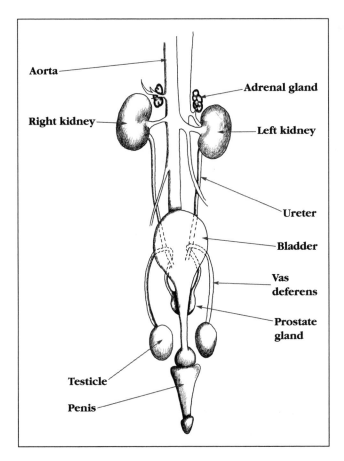

1-2 Male reproductive system

of the year. Most cats cycle in the early spring and to a lesser extent in the early fall. Although the majority of cats cycle in the spring and fall, some cats may come into heat at any time of the year. During the peak breeding times (spring and fall) the female cat will have multiple heats within a period of several months. *Polyestrus* is the term used to define multiple heats within a short span of time. Because the heat cycles in the cat tend to correspond with the spring and fall seasons, the cat is said to be "seasonally polyestrus."

Most female cats reach puberty and have their first heat cycle between five and nine months of age. Occasionally, one encounters a four-month-old cat that is sexually mature and capable of becoming pregnant. Persians as a breed are considered late maturers and may not reach puberty until one and a half years of age.

The estrous heat cycle of the female cat is divided into several stages: anestrus, proestrus, estrus and metestrus.

Anestrus is the term used to describe the quiescent (inactive) phase of the estrous cycle. This would be the period of no sexual activity. In most areas of the United States this would run from late September through mid-January. The low light factor, or short length of daylight, is a primary factor in reducing the heat cycles during the winter months. Cats kept indoors may be stimulated to cycle from artificial light sources for several weeks because these light levels are similar to those experienced during the peak breeding seasons of early spring and fall.

Proestrus is the term used to describe the stage of estrous immediately following anestrus. This is best described as the period where the cat is coming into heat, but is not yet in heat. The egg follicles of the ovaries are growing and maturing in preparation for the upcoming heat cycle and anticipated ovulation. Hormones such as the follicle stimulating hormone (FSH) and estrogen help promote the egg development occurring during this phase. Proestrus lasts about four days.

Estrus is the period of the heat cycle where the cat is able to become pregnant. It usually lasts 10 to 14 days. It is during this period that the owner may notice behavioral and other physical changes in the female. Hormones greatly influence the cat's behavior at this point. The cat "in heat" will vocalize and urinate frequently. Additionally, she will appear overly passionate by rolling, rubbing and assuming the breeding posture with the head and forelegs low to the ground and the rump area held high. Unlike the female dog, the female cat usually has little if any noticeable vaginal discharge in either the proestrus or estrus phase.

The actual breeding or intercourse takes place during the estrus phase. Intercourse usually lasts 10 seconds or less, but although the intercourse time is short, most females will breed repeatedly over a 24 to 48 hour period helping to assure a pregnancy. The act of breeding stimulates the female to ovulate or release eggs. This is termed induced ovulation. Contrast this to canines and humans where ovulation occurs even if intercourse does not. A cat not bred, and therefore not induced to ovulate, will usually go out of heat within 10 to 14 days. Because the cat was not induced to ovulate by a breeding, she will come into heat every two to three weeks until a breeding occurs or the breeding season passes.

It is possible to artificially induce ovulation in the cat. A rectal thermometer can be lightly inserted into the vagina to simulate penile penetration; this induces ovulation and therefore a cessation of the heat cycle. This ovulated, but not bred female usually will not cycle until the next breeding season, either spring or fall.

The time immediately after estrus is termed the **metestrus** period. The female will not pay attention or accept the male at this time.

DISORDERS OF THE FEMALE NOT DIRECTLY ASSOCIATED WITH PREGNANCY

VAGINITIS

Vaginitis refers to an inflammation or infection of the vagina. This may be the result of infectious agents such as bacteria and yeasts. More common than infections, however, are inflammations due to injury during breeding or birthing. Infections of the uterus (pyometra) and bladder (cystitis) may also involve the vagina since both the uterus and bladder ultimately empty into the vagina.

What Are the Symptoms?
Usually a slight, but visibly apparent vaginal discharge is noted as a result of vaginitis. The cat's excessive licking and grooming of the vaginal opening may obscure the discharge, however. As a result of the excessive licking, the vulva may actually become irritated causing redness, swelling and hair loss about the area.

What Are the Risks?
The majority of cases involving vaginitis are not serious. In fact, many cats self-limit this behavior with no treatment necessary. However, advanced cases of vaginitis can be very painful, and infections may spread to other areas such as the uterus. Untreated infections can be very serious and, in some instances, life threatening.

What Is the Treatment?
Treatment depends on the exact cause. Oral antibiotics are used if bacteria are involved. Vaginal flushes, or douches, are occasionally used to flush the vagina and help eliminate bacteria, yeasts and other infectious agents.

OVARIAN CYSTS

Occasionally, just as in humans, cysts can grow on or within the ovaries of the female cat. One or both ovaries may become cystic. Cysts are small fluid-filled, "blister-like" swellings on the ovary tissue. Ovarian cysts may actually produce hormones and prolong the female's heat cycles. This may create excessive breeding tendencies usually referred to as nymphomania.

What Are the Symptoms?
There are usually no outward signs of ovarian cysts. Many are discovered incidentally during abdominal surgeries or through skilled

palpations. As mentioned, sometimes ovarian cysts will create hormone imbalances that cause prolonged heat cycles and nymphomania.

What Are the Risks?
From a medical standpoint ovarian cysts are not serious. They can, however, disrupt breeding cycles and can be a cause of infertility in the breeding queen.

What Is the Treatment?
The best treatment to eliminate ovarian cysts is an ovariohysterectomy (spay), which removes the ovaries and uterus. Medical therapy, including hormone treatments, has not been very successful in treating ovarian cysts. Medical therapy is generally *not* recommended.

PYOMETRA

Pyometra is a disease of the uterus caused by an accumulation of purulent material (pus) within the uterus. If the opening into the cervix is closed, the purulent material can not drain out through the vagina, but stays confined to the cervix. This is sometimes referred to as a *closed pyometra*. If the cervix is open and the infection does drain out through the vagina, this is referred to as an *open pyometra*.

The exact cause of a pyometra in the cat is not clearly understood. Female hormones such as progesterone and estrogen are definitely involved, but not thought to be the primary cause. Excessive levels of progesterones will stimulate the uterine wall glands to oversecrete and perhaps become cystic.

Excessive levels of estrogens cause the cervix to open. This allows bacteria into the vagina and then the uterus. The vagina is exposed to the outside; therefore disease-causing bacteria are commonly present in the vagina, but not the uterus. The bacteria *E. coli* is the most common bacteria isolated from cats with a pyometra.

Once bacteria enter the uterus and cause a pyometra, the accumulation of pus and uterine secretions begins to build. The normal cat uterus has uterine horns about six inches long and the diameter of a normal shoelace. With a pyometra the uterine horns and body enlarge to about the size of a human thumb in diameter and up to ten inches in length (see figure 1-3). In a sense, the uterus acts like a big infected abscess within the abdomen.

What Are the Symptoms?
Although the uterus becomes greatly enlarged, it is deep within the abdomen so enlargement is not easily recognized by the owner. The abdomen may appear slightly enlarged and tense. In an open-ended

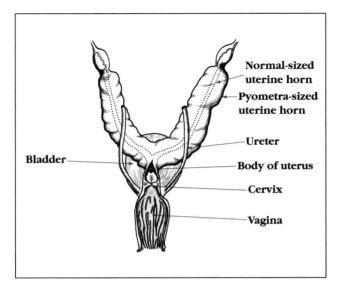

1-3   Pyometra

pyometra a sticky, yellow vaginal discharge may be present. Most cats with either an open or closed pyometra will lick the vulva area excessively, perhaps in an attempt to alleviate the pain. As the pyometra worsens the patient will outwardly appear ill. Toxins from the infected uterus will inhibit kidney function and many cats will appear excessively thirsty. Most become anorexic and will vomit. A fever may or may not be present.

What Are the Risks?

A pyometra is serious and life threatening. Most cats become acutely ill within several days of the onset of symptoms. Any suspected case of pyometra is a medical emergency and a veterinarian should be contacted without delay. *If left untreated the uterus may eventually rupture causing bacteria and pus to enter the abdomen and other organs. A ruptured pyometra is generally fatal,* occasionally even with aggressive medical therapy.

What Is the Treatment?

The best treatment for pyometra is an ovariohysterectomy (spay) to remove the infected uterus. Mild, early-detected cases have been treated with antibiotics to some degree of success. Hormone therapy has been used in some patients in an attempt to open the cervix in a closed pyometra to allow the uterus to drain. This therapy, coupled with antibiotics and uterine flushes, has helped save reproductive capabilities in valuable breeding animals. Medical treatment by any method is successful only in about 10 percent of all cases. Its usage is limited to valuable breeding queens in which an ovariohysterectomy (spay) is to be avoided.

CYSTIC ENDOMETRIAL HYPERPLASIA

Occasionally the glands lining the uterine wall become enlarged and develop cysts resembling water-filled sacs. This is called cystic endometrial hyperplasia.

What Are the Symptoms?
No outward symptoms are usually noticed by the owner. Infertility or failure to get pregnant may be possible signs in the breeding queen. The uterus may feel enlarged when palpated by the trained hand.

What Are the Risks?
Most patients with cystic endometrial hyperplasia live normal lives. They may, however, have abnormal estrous cycles (heats) and have reproduction failures as a result of an abnormal uterus.

What Is the Treatment?
The treatment is an ovariohysterectomy (spay), which removes the ovaries as well as the abnormal uterus.

CHRONIC ENDOMETRITIS

Chronic endometritis refers to an infection of the uterine lining that has persisted at a low level over a long period of time (weeks to months). Bacteria remain in the uterus and cause a mild infection. There is no large accumulation of pus and toxins as is the case with a pyometra. (Please see page 6.) *E. coli* is the most common bacteria associated with a chronic endometritis.

What Are the Symptoms?
Most cats have no signs recognizable by the owner. Breeding queens will fail to have healthy kittens. Abortions, stillbirths and early kitten death are all common. Occasionally a few kittens will survive and develop normally.

What Are the Risks?
Many patients are normal, but they experience repeated reproductive failures. Failure to get pregnant, inability to cycle, abortions, stillborns, infant deaths and small litters are all associated with this disorder. The mother, however, usually appears normal unless complications develop from dead or aborted fetuses.

What Is the Treatment?

Aggressive antibiotic therapy, usually for two to four weeks is indicated. Occasionally in identified breeding individuals, antibiotics are administered beginning two weeks prior to birthing and continued for one week into the lactation period. In unresponsive patients, ovariohysterectomy (spay) is the surgical treatment of choice. This removes the infected uterus and ovaries.

ACUTE METRITIS

An acute metritis is the sudden onset of a uterine infection. It is much more severe than the low-grade chronic endometritis. It usually occurs after the estrous cycle as a result of bacteria entering the uterus through the open cervix. It is also common following artificial insemination with non-sterile instruments. It may also occur after birthing, especially after a prolonged or difficult labor. Regardless of its cause, the end result is that bacteria such as *E. coli, staphylococci* and/or *streptococci* have been allowed to enter the uterus and cause rapid onset of infection.

What Are the Symptoms?

Because the infection is severe, the pregnant mother will usually fail to care for the litter once it arrives. She will not groom herself or the kittens. She may abandon the kittens, in which case they may die. The affected cat, whether bred or not, will develop a fever, vomit and become anorexic. A thick, reddish-brown, foul-smelling vaginal discharge is usually noted.

What Are the Risks?

An acute metritis is serious and life threatening to the cat. The kittens, if present, may succumb due to neglect unless they are hand-raised. Bacteria may also enter the mammary glands and milk posing a risk to the kittens. Left untreated, a cat with acute metritis will usually die.

What Is the Treatment?

Aggressive oral antibiotic therapy to kill the offending bacteria is necessary. Flushing of the vagina and uterus with antibiotic solutions is indicated. Intravenous fluids will be necessary if the queen is dehydrated. If medical therapy fails, then an ovariohysterectomy (spay) should be performed to remove the ovaries and infected uterus.

MAMMARY CANCER—BREAST CANCER

Mammary cancer occasionally occurs in the cat, but not as frequently as it does in dogs and humans.

The tumor type can be either a "mixed mammary" (in which many different cell types are present) or an adenocarcinoma (a tumor rising from glandular cells). Regardless of the type, these may spread via the lymph glands to other sites of the body.

The tumor rarely, if ever, occurs in females that have been spayed at an early age. It is thought that the tumor is stimulated or brought on by one or more of the female hormones associated with heat cycles, specifically estrogen. These hormones are produced and released by the ovaries, which are removed in a spay.

Mammary tumors are not usually seen until the animal is six or more years of age (see figure 1-4). Some cats will have several different

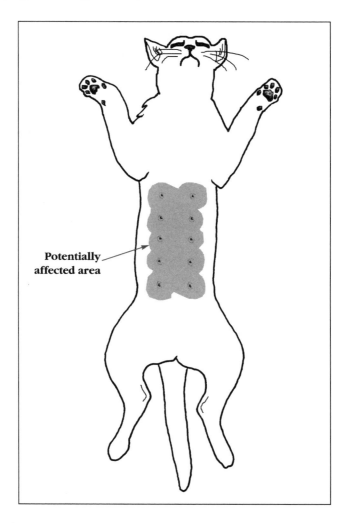

Potentially affected area

1-4　Breast cancer

tumors developing within various glands simultaneously. They develop slowly, but exhibit rapid periods of growth, both in size and numbers, immediately following heat cycles.

What Are the Symptoms?
Mammary tumors are easily felt through the skin. They are very hard, round masses with an irregular or bumpy surface. Sometimes they are close to the surface, lying just under the skin. At this location on a cat with white or very light-colored skin, the tumors can be seen and have a light-yellow color. Although they can be found in any of the mammary glands, they are most frequently noted in the two rear ones.

Usually there are no clinical signs associated with mammary tumors, unless they drain or spread to other parts of the body. Sometimes these tumors grow rapidly, rupture out through the skin over the mammary gland and drain a pink-tinged fluid. These are usually malignant tumors that spread to other parts of the body; their presence can be detected from the effects they cause on other structures. A common example of this would be when they spread to the lungs and cause a cough or difficult respiration.

What Are the Risks?
The vast majority of all mammary tumors are malignant and if left untreated will threaten the life of the patient. They typically spread via the lymph vessels to the lungs, and from there to many other organs. At these sites they replace or destroy tissue that is necessary for life.

What Is the Treatment?
Once tumors are encountered, the best treatment is surgical removal. If this is done early in the course of the disease, the cancer may be eliminated before it has a chance to spread to other areas of the body.

DISORDERS OF THE FEMALE AS A RESULT OF PREGNANCY, BIRTHING AND LACTATION

ECTOPIC PREGNANCY

It is not uncommon for the breeding queen to develop an ectopic pregnancy. This is an instance where the fertilized egg fails to properly enter the oviduct and instead implants outside the uterus, usually in the abdominal cavity wall.

What Are the Symptoms?

There are no outward symptoms. Usually the breeding female simply returns to heat during the time in which she should have been pregnant.

What Are the Risks?

Ectopic pregnancies pose little risk to the mother. The fetus dies at an early stage and is usually reabsorbed or walled off with scar tissue. A palpable mass can occasionally be felt in the abdomen.

What Is the Treatment?

No treatment is usually required. Spaying the affected queen prevents future occurrences. At the time of surgery the dead fetal mass can be removed.

DYSTOCIA

Difficulty in delivering the kittens is termed dystocia. This can occur when the mother is unable to push the kitten through the birth canal or the delivery simply takes too long. It has many causes.

The problem may relate to the fetus. When there is only one or very few kittens, they will typically be larger than normal and have difficulty getting through the birth canal. In other cases, the alignment of a kitten in relation to the opening of the cervix may cause problems if a kitten is malaligned. This is termed an "abnormal presentation." That is, instead of pointing directly or straight through the canal, their heads may be bent backward or they might be coming out sideways. In kittens, it is not considered abnormal if the kitten comes "tail or rear quarters first;" probably 45 percent of all feline births occur in this manner.

In some instances, dystocia may be caused by an abnormal structure in the mother. Her bony pelvis may be too small to allow the kittens to pass through. This can be a conformational abnormality or the result of an injury. In other cases, her uterus may fail to contract correctly (see "Uterine Inertia," page 13). This is common when the kittens are smaller than normal and, as a result, inadequate uterine dilation fails to stimulate contractions. Behavior problems are also noted in first time mothers. They may resist straining because of the pain, fear or simply lack of experience.

What Are the Risks?

Dystocia frequently leads to fetal death. Extreme pressure during prolonged periods of uterine contraction can severely damage fragile, young kittens. Additionally, this pressure from being within the birth canal for too long can impede circulation of oxygen-rich blood through the umbilical cord to the kitten. If the neonate cannot get oxygen while in the birth canal, it quickly suffocates.

If the kitten cannot be expelled by the mother, dystocia may also result in her death. This can occur immediately or over a period of several days because of the huge mass of decaying fetal tissue trapped within her body.

What Is the Treatment?

Dystocia is always a medical emergency. Anytime that a queen has had consistent contractions for more than three hours before the first kitten is born or for more than one hour for any subsequent one, the queen should be seen immediately by a veterinarian. He or she may be able to "pull" the kitten with the use of medical instruments and help the efforts of the queen through medications such as oxytocin. In more severe situations, a caesarean section can be performed.

UTERINE INERTIA

A unique form of dystocia is uterine inertia. In this condition, the uterus either fails to initiate contractions or stops prematurely. This prevents the normal expulsion of the kittens.

This can have several different causes. In cats, as the number of fetuses within a litter increases, their individual size decreases (and vice versa). Because of large litters and small kittens, the uterus is not as dilated as it would ordinarily be.

One of the major factors stimulating the uterine contractions is the degree of uterine dilation. Therefore, with small kittens, it is easily understood why uterine inertia is more common. Some queens have repeated problems with each pregnancy. In these it is thought to be an individual or genetic trait.

Uterine inertia can occur in any queen, especially during a prolonged and difficult birthing (kindling). In these cases, it is believed that the uterine muscles or the animal in general simply becomes exhausted.

What Are the Symptoms?

Classically, in cases of uterine inertia, the female simply goes out of "labor" prematurely. There will be kittens present within the uterus, but she makes no further effort to expel them. Kittens already born are treated normally.

What Are the Risks?

If the fetuses are not born within 24 to 36 hours after the beginning of labor, they can be expected to die. If they are not discovered and are left within the mother, she will rapidly become ill and may also die. She simply cannot tolerate or deal with such a large mass of dead or dying tissue within her body.

What Is the Treatment?

When diagnosed, medications such as oxytocin may be useful to stimulate uterine contractions. However, if estrogen, the naturally produced hormone associated with birthing, is no longer at significant levels within the body, oxytocin usually fails to function. In these cases only a caesarean section can be performed to correct the situation. Queens known to have problems with uterine inertia are usually X-rayed or ultrasounded late in the pregnancy to determine the number of fetuses so that therapy can be initiated as soon as the first signs of the disorder are observed.

UTERINE PROLAPSE

Uterine prolapse occurs when the vagina and vulva are penetrated by one or both uterine horns. The most common time for this to occur is immediately and up to 48 hours after birthing. It rarely happens before all of the kittens have been born.

What Are the Symptoms?

The symptoms are obvious as the bright pink to red uterus appears like a sausage(s) hanging from the vulva.

What Are the Risks?

A prolapsed uterus is serious and should be treated immediately. Left untreated the blood supply to the uterus is constricted and tissue is destroyed. This can lead to life-threatening infections.

What Is the Treatment?

If treated early, the uterus can be put back in place. An anesthesia may be required. In severe cases, the uterus may need to be surgically repositioned. If a queen experiences more than one uterine prolapse, it is generally recommended to perform an ovariohysterectomy (spay).

RETAINED PLACENTAS (FETAL MEMBRANES)

There is always great concern by cat owners regarding retained placentas. During the birth process called "kindling" in the cat ("whelping" in the dog), fetal membranes (placentas) are expulsed from the vagina at random. There may be several kittens born before the first placenta is passed. Quite commonly it is difficult to actually count the expulsed placentas as some pass together or are eaten by the mother before they can be detected by the owner. If the placentas remain within the uterus they are said to be "retained." Although much written about, retained fetal membranes in the cat are not commonly encountered by the authors.

What Are the Symptoms?
If the placenta(s) has been retained after kindling, the most noticeable sign is a brownish-red discharge from the vulva. The cat will usually lick excessively about the area.

What Are the Risks?
If only a little fetal tissue is retained, it may go unnoticed and not present a problem. It is possible for the queen to develop a low grade chronic endometritis (see page 8) leading to possible fertility problems.

What Is the Treatment?
Treatment varies widely. If the patient is not a valuable breeding queen, the treatment of choice is an ovariohysterectomy (spay) to remove the ovaries and affected uterus. Drugs such as ergonovine maleate have been used to stimulate uterine shrinkage and membrane expulsion. Antibiotics are used to treat infections if present.

PROLONGED UTERINE HEMORRHAGE FOLLOWING BIRTH

It is normal for the queen to pass blood from the vulva for up to five days after giving birth. If bleeding persists beyond five days it is considered prolonged. The most common cause of a prolonged hemorrhage is due to improper uterine shrinkage (involution) of the uterus once the fetuses have passed. It is normal for vessels within the uterine wall to bleed (hemorrhage) once the fetuses detach and are born. If the uterus shrinks or constricts properly to its normal non-pregnant size, the bleeding vessels are constricted and the hemorrhaging stops. If the uterus doesn't constrict in a timely fashion (three to five days), then the bleeding continues.

What Are the Symptoms?
Bright red blood discharging from the mother's vulva longer than five days following birthing is the main sign. The kittens will all be normal.

What Are the Risks?
Assuming that the bleeding is due to the failure of the uterus to constrict, there are few, if any risks to the animal with this condition. In

some cases, the occurrence or regularity of future heat cycles may be affected. It is important to eliminate from the diagnosis other possible disorders such as cancer or a blood clotting disorder.

What Is the Treatment?
In most cases, this condition resolves itself. If necessary, treatments using ergonovine are believed to be the most effective. Many feel that injections of oxytocin in the first 24 hours following birthing may prevent or lessen the possibility of this disorder occurring.

MAMMARY HYPERPLASIA

Mammary hyperplasia refers to an enlargement of the mammary glands in the non-pregnant cat. It most frequently occurs after the estrous (heat) cycle, especially in young cats following their *first* cycle. It is believed that higher-than-normal levels of estrogen are the cause.

What Are the Symptoms?
The mammary glands enlarge, become painful and may provide a brownish discharge from the nipples. The glands, in addition to becoming painful, will feel warm to the touch.

What Are the Risks?
This is not an infection, but rather a hormone imbalance. It will usually subside, but is likely to reoccur after future estrous cycles. It is not life threatening.

What Is the Treatment?
Because it is likely to reoccur after every heat cycle, it is best if prone patients are spayed to remove the ovaries and uterus. Diuretics such as Lasix may be used to shrink the mammary glands to reduce swelling and pain.

MASTITIS

Mastitis is an infection of the mammary glands that is usually caused by bacteria. This commonly occurs in felines during lactation and is quite rare at other times. It is possible that bacteria gain access to the breast tissue through the bloodstream being carried there from infections elsewhere in the body. However, it is believed that in most cases the bacteria enter the mammary gland by migrating through the nipple opening during or following nursing. The organisms present are those commonly found on the skin or normally passed in the stools of the cat.

The bacteria *staphylococcus* and *streptococcus* are the most common pathogens.

What Are the Symptoms?

At any one time mastitis will usually be found only in one or two of the mammary glands. The last two or three glands on either side will be the ones most frequently affected. The infected glands will initially become hard and in a few hours to a day become swollen, hot, discolored (from red to dark blue) and very painful to the touch.

The cat will have a fever and may go off food. Left untreated, the mastitis usually develops into an abscess that will rupture, draining a thick yellowish pus. In the cat, milk normally appears like a thin form of cow's milk. With mastitis, it becomes yellowish-white with obvious lumps and a foul smell. The toxic effects of the milk soon spread to the nursing kittens. They become lethargic, discontinue nursing, develop swollen abdomens and, in some cases, die. Some females will have repeated bouts of mastitis during future pregnancies, with every instance requiring treatment.

What Are the Risks?

Mastitis is a risk to both the queen and the nursing kittens. The infection and resulting abscess can spread to other parts of the mother's body. Some infected glands may become scarred to the extent that future milk production or nursing is impossible from that gland. In the kittens, it can be fatal, because they automatically consume large quantities of bacteria. At this stage of their lives, they have a very low level of resistance, and what starts out as an infection in the intestinal tract (enteritis) quickly spreads throughout their bodies.

What Is the Treatment?

Mastitis must be treated immediately. If it is first observed in the evening, the cat should be taken to the veterinarian on an emergency basis rather than waiting for the following day. If milk and the infected discharge can still be expressed through the nipple, as much as possible should be "milked out." If an abscess has formed or the gland is impacted, it is usually necessary to lance the infected gland and drain its contents. In some cases, in addition to oral antibiotics, it may be necessary to flush out the infected area for several days with an antibacterial solution or ointment. This cleanses the area and prevents it from healing over, which would result in the formation of another abscess.

The animal is placed on a broad-spectrum antibiotic, and supportive care is given as needed. Problem queens have repeated bouts of mastitis in subsequent pregnancies. These animals may be placed on antibiotics in a preventative fashion throughout lactation.

Kittens are usually removed from their mother and supplemented with milk replacers until the queen's milk appears normal. Antibiotics are frequently also given to the kittens.

ECLAMPSIA (LACTATIONAL TETANY OR MILK FEVER)

This disease of nursing queens typically occurs three to four weeks into lactation. It is the result of abnormally low calcium levels within the blood. Some cat health experts believe that the calcium levels are depressed by the production of milk and the development of the fetal skeletons. Additionally, many believe that it may be further exaggerated by low calcium levels in the diet or poor absorption of this mineral in the gut.

This condition may be caused by any or all of these factors and is further affected by hormones and genetics. For whatever reason, during this period the blood calcium levels may drop rapidly, bringing on a life-threatening situation. It is most common in queens with four or more nursing kittens as they consume large quantities of milk and deplete the queen's calcium levels.

What Are the Symptoms?
Early in the syndrome, affected queens may do little more than appear uneasy or anxious. They will fidget, often bouncing back and forth to their kittens. As this condition progresses, the animal will become more distressed, exhibiting heavy panting and moaning as if in pain. From this point the signs become more physical, with muscle twitching and staggering. The animal may walk peg-legged, and there can be drooling and diarrhea. In a few hours these signs can further elevate to seizures, extremely rapid heart rates and death.

What Are the Risks?
Most cases of eclampsia are progressive. As the kittens continue to nurse, the blood calcium levels continue to drop. Calcium is necessary for muscle and nerve function. As the calcium levels decrease, the coordination between neural transmission and muscular activity is lost. This results in uncontrolled muscular activity ranging from mild twitching to uncontrollable convulsions.

As the condition progresses, the heart muscles and those responsible for breathing become involved. These muscles are obviously necessary for life, and as they lose their ability to function, the animal can easily die.

What Is the Treatment?

Treatment for eclampsia must be initiated as soon as possible. Although the condition is life threatening, it is easy to treat. Initially, intravenous injections of calcium are given. These usually eliminate the clinical signs associated with the disease immediately. However, treatment using oral or subcutaneous injections of calcium products usually continues through the remainder of the lactation. In severe cases, the kittens may be removed from the mother and fed milk replacers.

Queens that have had a problem with eclampsia are usually treated in a preventative fashion for future litters. They may have calcium supplements added to their diet during pregnancy, and these will be continued through the entire nursing period.

DISORDERS OF THE MALE REPRODUCTIVE SYSTEM

PARAPHIMOSIS (DUE TO HAIR RING)

The penis of the male has about 120 small "spike-like" projections on the surface. When a tomcat breeds a female, hair from the female may accumulate on the spikes of the male's penis much like human hair on a hairbrush. The accumulated hair wraps around the penis and may prevent it from being retracted back inside its protective sheath. The extended penis with an inability to retract is termed paraphimosis.

What Are the Symptoms?

An affected tomcat will typically behave as if he is still mounting the female. He may excessively lick about the penile area in an attempt to remove the hair.

What Are the Risks?

Accumulated hair on the penis usually presents no great health problem, but it can interfere with breeding. Most tomcats simply remove the hair by grooming after the breeding has subsided.

What Is the Treatment?

Usually no treatment is needed as the male cat is capable of removing the hair. In order not to delay breeding, however, the hair can be manually removed with forceps.

ORCHITIS

Orchitis refers to an inflammation or infection of the testicles. It is not common to have bacteria affect the teste(s) of the cat. Orchitis warrants no further discussion here.

CRYPTORCHIDISM

The normal kitten is born with both testicles already inside the scrotum. Occasionally, one or both testicles fail to descend and remain within the abdominal cavity or musculature. If only one testicle is retained, this is called monorchidism. If the testicle(s) is not descended by birth, it should be by six months of age. If they do not descend, then the kitten is a cryptorchid, or monorchid if it has one descended testicle. Occasionally a testicle will move back and forth from the scrotum to the abdominal musculature. This is called a "yo-yo" testis.

What Are the Symptoms?
The main symptom is the absence of one or both testicles in the scrotal sac. If neither testicle descends they remain small and inactive, therefore producing reduced amounts of the male hormone testosterone. This may result in a feminized appearance of the tom. The glands about the jowl area will be smaller than those of a normal tomcat. Females have smaller glands and their head appears thinner; the same is true of cryptorchids.

What Are the Risks?
The main risk associated with retained testicles is that they are prone to developing cancer. *Cancer* of the testicles is not *common* in normal or cryptorchid cats, but is *more likely* to occur in cryptorchids. In general, testicular cancer is considerably less common in cats than in dogs.

What Is the Treatment?
Usually, abdominal surgery is performed to remove the testicle(s) within the abdomen or its muscles. This prevents all possibility of testicular cancer. It should be noted that monorchids, those with one testicle in the scrotum, are fertile. Although not recommended in a breeding program, they can reproduce. Cryptorchids, those with no testicles in the scrotum, are sterile.

CHAPTER 2

The Mouth, Teeth, Gums and Salivary Glands

Food enters the digestive tract through the mouth. The upper and lower jaws are lined with teeth that are used for tearing and shredding food. The **infant** feline has **26 teeth** while the **adult** mouth contains **30 teeth.** The exact number can vary slightly (see figure 2-1). The salivary glands produce saliva, which mixes with the food in the mouth. Saliva acts as a lubricant, plus it contains ptyalin, an enzyme that helps break down starch that is in the diet.

The **teeth** are living tissues. The outer layer is made up of enamel, the hardest substance in the feline body (see figure 2-2). Dentine is the middle layer; the core is called the pulp. The pulp contains nerves and blood vessels that nourish the tooth. The root of the tooth is buried beneath the gum. Some teeth, such as incisors, have one root while the others, such as the upper fourth premolars, have as many as three roots.

The feline has four pairs of **salivary glands** (see figure 2-3). The parotid, mandibular, sublingual and zygomatic glands are all paired and produce saliva. Each gland has its own duct to carry saliva from the gland to the mouth cavity.

The **tongue** of the feline is a useful and complex organ. It is used to manipulate food about the mouth and allows the animal to drink water. The tongue's taste buds recognize flavors, aid in cleaning the body and communicate with other pets.

When a feline drinks, liquid is transported on top of the tongue and into the mouth. This is called lapping. Contrast this to the canine who carries liquid under the tongue in a gulping fashion. A cat is relatively silent when drinking, whereas a canine must repeatedly thrust the tongue into water to gulp. When water is gulped, much air can be

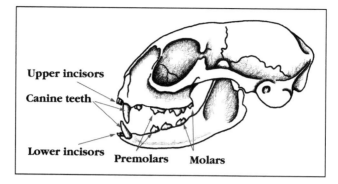

2-1   Feline toothed skull

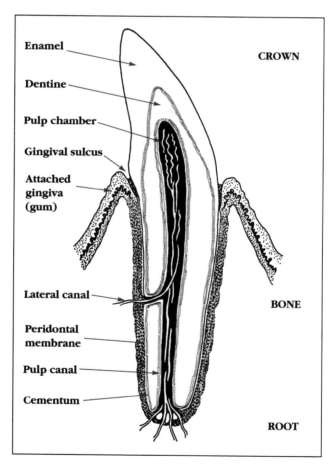

2-2   Tooth detail

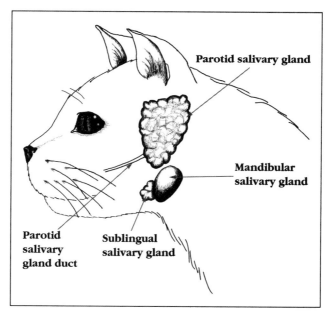

2-3 Salivary glands

transported along with the liquid. This makes hiccups a common occurrence in puppies, but not in kittens who lap their liquids. The feline tongue is also an organ of grooming. On its dorsal surface are cornified barb-like structures that act like a comb to help cleanse the hair coat (see figure 2-4).

The gums of the feline are normally pink in coloration; however, it is not uncommon for some cats to develop dark spots or pigmented areas about their lips and mouth. Orange or yellow cats have the highest incidence of pigment spots about their mouth. These develop with age and are normal.

RETAINED BABY (DECIDUOUS) TEETH

By four weeks of age kittens usually get their deciduous teeth, commonly known as baby teeth. Most kittens have 26 deciduous teeth. Beginning around four months of age the deciduous teeth are replaced by the bigger and stronger permanent teeth. It takes an additional three to five months for all of the permanent teeth to replace the baby teeth. The adult feline averages 30 permanent teeth.

Occasionally the permanent teeth do not erupt immediately under the deciduous teeth and therefore do not force the baby teeth out. When a pet has both an adult and baby tooth at the same site, the

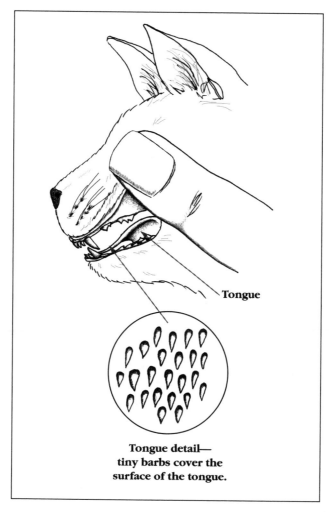

Tongue

Tongue detail—
tiny barbs cover the
surface of the tongue.

2-4   Cat tongue

problem is referred to as a retained deciduous tooth. In the feline it is usually the incisors or baby canine teeth that are retained.

What Are the Symptoms?

Commonly an extra set, or double row, of teeth is noted. In the case of the large canine teeth it is usually the upper deciduous ones that are retained. The permanent canine teeth typically erupt in front of the deciduous canine (see figure 2-5).

What Are the Risks?

Retained baby teeth frequently cause a crowding of the teeth along the gum line. This crowding displaces the permanent teeth and causes them to grow at odd angles. The development of the bones of the jaw can also be affected as the abnormal placement of the teeth interfere with normal growth. Retained teeth may also die and abscess, causing infections of the mouth to develop.

What Is the Treatment?
All abnormally retained deciduous teeth should be extracted. This will usually require anesthesia and surgical extraction. Check a kitten's mouth weekly until about seven months of age for abnormal teeth. Consult with a veterinarian for an oral examination if any retained teeth are suspected.

DENTAL CARIES

Cavities (or caries) are corrosions through the tooth enamel. This demineralization or loss of tooth structure is commonly the result of bacterial or chemical action upon the tooth surfaces.

What Are the Symptoms?
Cavities in teeth generally appear as dark areas on the surface of the tooth. A crater-like hole will usually develop and will vary in size depending on how long the cavity has been present.

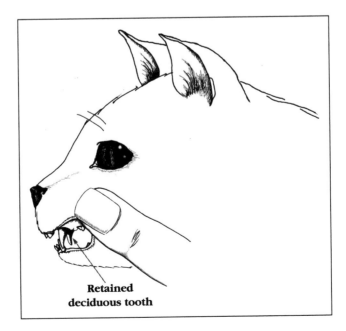

**Retained
deciduous tooth**

2-5 Retained tooth

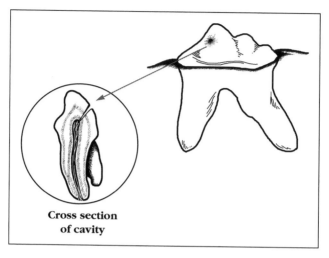

Cross section
of cavity

2-6 Cavity in tooth

What Are the Risks?

Probably because of low sugar diets, severe cavities are unusual in the feline. Most patients with cavities go untreated, and in many cases, even unnoticed. Cavities can, however, extend into the deeper pulp areas (see figure 2-6) of the tooth and cause pain or even kill the tooth.

What Is the Treatment?

As in humans, dental caries can be repaired to stop the progression. Veterinary dental techniques have improved significantly over the past decade, and veterinarians specializing in dental care are widely available. Cavities can now be drilled, cleaned and filled. In the past these teeth were simply extracted.

ABSCESSED TOOTH ROOTS

Sometimes the roots of teeth become infected. This is usually the result of gum disease where bacteria enters from the mouth and moves beneath the gum line causing an infection by the tooth roots. Any tooth can be involved, although most frequently the incisors, canines and the upper fourth premolars are the ones involved.

What Are the Symptoms?

Usually, a notable swelling is seen along the gum line where the tooth root embeds. If the abscess is draining into the mouth, a foul odor may be detected in the breath. In severe abscesses of tooth roots, a swelling may even be noticed on the face. Incisors simply become loose and fall

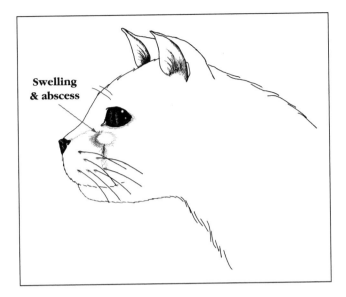

2-7   Abscessed tooth roots

out. Infected canine teeth may drain out the nasal passages and cause a large marble-size swelling or abscess on the muzzle. Abscesses of the upper fourth premolar are common in the feline. The fourth premolar has three roots that extend up under the eye. Commonly, the first indication of a root abscess is a swelling and/or drainage of the face immediately under the eye (see figure 2-7).

What Are the Risks?
Infected teeth are serious and cause great pain to the animal. Frequently because of the pain, the patient is unable to chew and will refuse to eat. If they do eat they will typically avoid chewing on the affected side. Untreated, the teeth die and are lost.

What Is the Treatment?
Antibiotic therapy alone is usually not enough to clear up the infection. In some cases the infected teeth are simply extracted, exposing the abscess and allowing it to drain. Root canals can be done in an effort to save the tooth. This is preferred, but more expensive. Antibiotic therapy is recommended following extraction.

FRACTURED TEETH

Fractured teeth in the feline are uncommon. Unlike their canine counterparts, cats do not chew on hard objects such as rocks or fencing, which can cause wear or cracking (fracture) of the teeth. Fractured

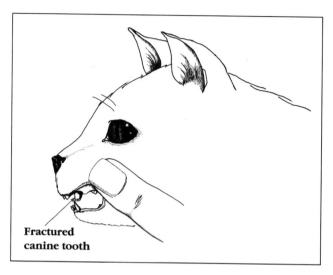

**Fractured
canine tooth**

2-8   Fractured tooth

teeth in the cat are usually the result of traumatic incidents such as automobile accidents. The most commonly fractured teeth are the long, "fang-like" canine teeth (see figure 2-8).

What Are the Symptoms?

Generally, the cracks or missing sections of teeth are fairly obvious. Routine examination of the mouth will help detect partial cracks. Following any injury to the head, the teeth should be carefully examined for cracks or missing sections.

What Are the Risks?

Fractures of the teeth often are not serious. Cracks that extend below the gum line or into the pulp may cause tooth death, however, and abscessation may result if the roots or pulp become exposed to bacteria.

What Is the Treatment?

If the animal is in pain from abscessation or a dead tooth, then extraction of the tooth is recommended. Specialized veterinary dentists can, in less severe cases, repair the fractures or even place an artificial crown upon the tooth much like in humans. These specialized procedures are more for cosmetic purposes than a medical necessity.

MALOCCLUSION OF THE TEETH

Malocclusion results when the upper teeth do not align properly with the lower teeth. Normally the teeth meet in a manner that allows powerful chewing and tearing of food. Teeth that do not align correctly are usually the result of abnormal jaw growth or malalignment of the teeth themselves.

What Are the Symptoms?
Oftentimes the malocclusion can only be visualized upon close examination of the teeth. Chewing abnormalities, such as food falling from the mouth, may be a symptom. The majority of malocclusion cases seen at our hospitals involve improper length of one or both jaws. If the lower jaw protrudes too far beyond the upper, the animal is said to be undershot. Sometimes this is referred to as a "salmon jaw." Conversely, if the upper jaw protrudes beyond the lower, the animal is said to be overshot. This is occasionally referred to as "parrot mouth."

What Are the Risks?
Malocclusion usually presents no great risk to the patient. The ingestion of food and chewing may be hindered somewhat, but most patients still perform these functions quite well. Tartar and plaque will build up excessively on teeth if abnormal wearing surfaces are created. Tooth wear can also be excessive if two teeth constantly grind upon each other. Patients with severely undershot jaws may have difficulty picking up food, and therefore larger chunks are more easily ingested than are smaller ones.

What Is the Treatment?
Most patients do not need to get the malocclusion treated. But if teeth wear excessively due to abnormal grinding, then extractions may be necessary. Teeth should be routinely brushed and cleaned to prevent the abnormal buildup of tartar and plaque. Veterinary dental specialists can be consulted if one desires to alter the malocclusion. This is occasionally done for cosmetic as well as medical reasons. *It is not wise to breed pets with malformed jaws as there is a hereditary link in most affected patients.*

GINGIVAL HYPERPLASIA

Occasionally, for reasons probably due to constant irritation, the cells of the gums will increase in size and number creating a cauliflowered or overgrown appearance. In some cases, viruses have been implicated as a possible cause of gingival hyperplasia.

What Are the Symptoms?
Small growths will arise from the gum tissue, usually along the tooth line. These areas of gum hypertrophy often resemble the head of a

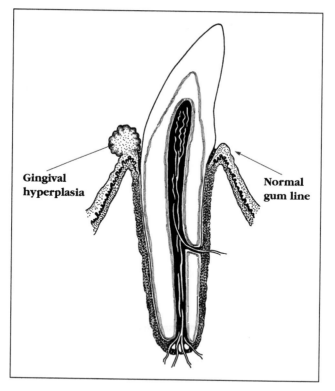

2-9 Gingival hyperplasia

cauliflower (see figure 2-9). The gums may bleed due to damage while chewing.

What Are the Risks?
A benign growth of cells, gingival hyperplasia poses no serious health threat. The gums may be damaged from chewing; they may bleed and become painful.

What Is the Treatment?
The areas of excessive tissue growth can be surgically removed. Anesthesia is generally required. If regrowth occurs then surgery may need to be repeated. The growth is usually biopsied and differentiated from more serious disorders such as cancer. Gingival hyperplasia is neither serious nor life threatening.

GINGIVITIS

Gingivitis describes an inflammation or infection of the gums. When plaque and tartar build up on the teeth, the gum areas that attach to the dirty teeth become loose and pull away from the teeth. The loose gums allow air and bacteria to enter the lower tissues, possibly down to the roots of the teeth.

What Are the Symptoms?

The gums will appear red or purplish and are usually swollen (see figure 2-10). A discharge is normally noted, with infected material draining from around the teeth giving them a slimy appearance. A foul breath is almost always present. Gingivitis should be a primary consideration in any case of bad breath.

As the gums swell and become painful, chewing difficulties or reluctance to eat may be noted. Excessive drooling may occur, and in cats (as opposed to dogs) it is not considered normal. Ulcers with bleeding may develop in advanced cases.

What Are the Risks?

Infected gums are more serious than often thought. As bacteria invade the gums and teeth, they can also enter the bloodstream and cause infection in more critical areas such as the heart. Additionally, bacteria

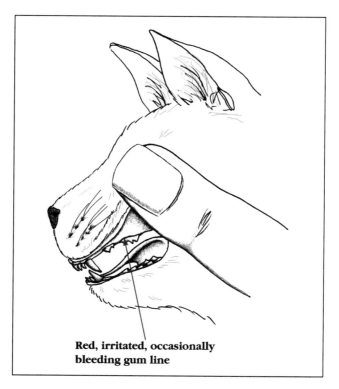

Red, irritated, occasionally bleeding gum line

2-10   Gingivitis

are constantly "showering" the larynx and trachea and being inhaled into the fragile lungs. Maintaining good oral hygiene is an important component of the overall health of the animal.

What Is the Treatment?

Rather than treating gingivitis, it is far better to practice good oral hygiene as a preventative. All cats should have their teeth cleaned and gums massaged by routine brushing. Excellent toothpastes and mouthwashes are now marketed specifically for pets. Used regularly, these products will greatly reduce gingivitis.

The diet can also be modified. Diets of dry food tend to be abrasive and help keep the teeth free of tartar and plaque. Routine examinations by veterinarians, coupled with prophylactic cleanings, are also recommended. Once developed, gingivitis is best treated with ultrasonic cleansing by a veterinarian. Some or all of the teeth may need to be removed depending on severity. Long-term antibiotic therapy is usually necessary to kill and control the disease-causing bacteria.

GLOSSITIS

An inflammation of the tongue is termed glossitis. Although tongue infections are rare, it is not uncommon for the tongue to become irritated or injured. Sources of irritation include burrs from weeds, bee stings and burns.

What Are the Symptoms?

Inflammations of the tongue are very painful, at least initially. Reluctance to eat is the most common sign associated with a glossitis. In the case of burrs, one may notice the "slivers" or splinters protruding from the surface of the tongue.

What Are the Risks?

The tongue tends to heal quickly even when severely damaged. Burrs must be removed before healing can begin.

What Is the Treatment?

Usually, no treatment is necessary. In the case of porcupine quills or burrs, the foreign material must be removed. Surgery is probably needed as most patients are not receptive to tongue manipulation. Antibiotics are often used to prevent infection from spreading elsewhere in the body.

TONSILLITIS

Tonsillitis describes an inflammation of the tonsils. Generally, the tonsils are considered part of the lymphatic system. Felines have two tonsils located on the sides of the oral cavity at the rear. They are each found within a fold of tissue referred to as a tonsilar crypt. When enlarged, they fold out of the crypt and are easily visible with the naked eye.

What Are the Symptoms?
As with other throat and mouth irritations, many patients will be reluctant to eat and will drool excessively because swallowing is painful. Other cats with the same condition will swallow repeatedly. The tonsils will appear enlarged and reddened.

What Are the Risks?
As in humans, tonsillitis is seldom serious; however, it can be chronic and annoying.

What Is the Treatment?
The cause of the enlarged tonsils should be determined. *Streptococcus* or other bacteria frequently infect the area. Foreign objects such as chicken bones lodged in the throat can cause inflammation of the tonsils. Antibiotics are effective if bacteria are the cause. Only in severe chronic tonsillitis of unknown origin should the tonsils be removed. The feline tonsils are lymphoid tissue and are therefore important in fighting diseases; when possible they should be left intact.

CLEFT PALATE

This is a skeletal disorder occasionally seen in kittens of all breeds. A cleft palate results when the bones forming the roof of the mouth do not grow normally. This results in an opening in the roof of the mouth that communicates into the nasal cavity.

What Are the Symptoms?
Kittens as young as one day old will often have milk come out of their noses as they nurse. They may also inhale milk into their lungs, causing a difficulty in breathing or even pneumonia. When the kitten's mouth is examined, a slit will be seen in the roof of the mouth.

What Are the Risks?

Most patients will die at an early age from pneumonia and/or malnourishment. The milk tends to enter the nasal passages and lungs rather than providing nourishment.

What Is the Treatment?

Mild openings in the mouth roof can be surgically corrected. More severe instances cannot. Frequently, if the cleft palate cannot be surgically closed, euthanasia is advised.

RODENT ULCER (EOSINOPHILIC GRANULOMA COMPLEX)

See Chapter 11, "The Skin, Hair and Nails."

TUMORS OF THE MOUTH

As with most areas of the body, the mouth tissues are susceptible to cancer. Fortunately, mouth cancer is not common in the feline. If stricken with cancer, however, the tumors may arise anywhere, including the gums, tongue, tonsils, palate and cheeks.

What Are the Symptoms?

Most patients with mouth cancer have a foul breath. Commonly the tumor(s) bleeds, sometimes profusely. As the tumor(s) grows, a reluctance to eat and weight loss will be noted. Excessive drooling is common. Upon oral examination most tumors can be visualized as growths larger than a marble.

What Are the Risks?

All cases of mouth cancer are serious. Most tumors found in this area are malignant. Many types will spread to other areas such as the lymph nodes or lungs.

What Is the Treatment?

Surgery to remove the cancerous growths is required. In some instances, chemotherapy and radiation treatments can be beneficial. Malignant tumors of the mouth commonly reoccur or spread to other areas despite treatment.

PICA—DEPRAVED APPETITE

PICA is a term used to describe a condition in which a patient eats objects not considered a normal part of the diet. Examples include pets that have an appetite for wood, sand, metal, stones, rubber, etc. PICA is not really a disorder of the mouth, but is rather a psychological abnormality. It is included here in case the objects are actually eaten.

What Are the Symptoms?
The symptoms simply include a history of eating objects undesirable for digestion. To have PICA, a patient generally does not just eat the objects once, but rather seems to be addicted to consuming the material.

What Are the Risks?
Eating foreign objects is risky in that many of these objects cannot pass normally through the gastrointestinal tract. Objects such as rocks and yarn can cause a blockage of the intestines requiring surgery to remove. Additionally, they may cause damage to the mouth or abnormal wear on the teeth.

What Is the Treatment?
Contrary to common belief, a patient with an abnormal appetite is not lacking in vitamins, minerals or any other nutrient. PICA is a psychlogical abnormality and is more a habit than a medical problem even though it can lead to such. There is no such cure for PICA; however, providing alternative edible objects and digestible treats will help.

It should be noted that eating grass is not considered a form of PICA; this behavior is normal for many cats. It is common for a cat to consume grass and occasionally vomit it back up. It is unknown why this happens, but it may be a method for wild cats to expel hairballs. Cats may also eat grass because of the juices it contains. Possibly, cats actually crave the taste of grass. Grass-eating is considered normal and is not an indicator of health such as intestinal parasites.

FOREIGN BODIES OF THE MOUTH

Felines occasionally get foreign bodies lodged in their mouths. Bones, sticks and strings are the most common. Poultry bones are common offenders.

What Are the Symptoms?
Drooling and gagging are the most noted symptoms. The cats aren't really gagging, but are manipulating the tongue in an attempt to remove the object. Commonly the objects are lodged across the upper palate between the teeth. String may wrap around the base of the

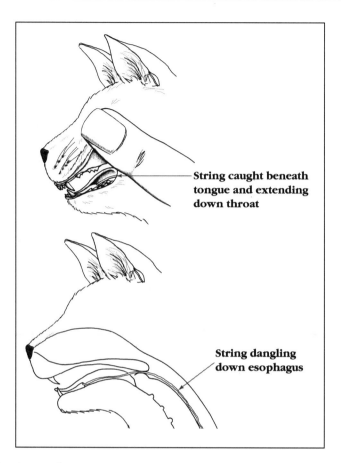

String caught beneath tongue and extending down throat

String dangling down esophagus

2-11   String in mouth

tongue (see figure 2-11) or be caught between the teeth. Bad breath will develop if the objects remain lodged. Many of these cats will not eat, while others go on as if nothing was wrong.

What Are the Risks?
If not promptly removed, the objects may cause infections of the gums and other structures. Many patients fail to eat and lose weight.

What Is the Treatment?
Treatment involves identifying and removing the object. Always examine around and under the tongue for pieces of string or similar material. String can loop under the tongue with the ends actually being swallowed into the stomach and intestines. Look closely, as string or fishing line may be difficult to see. Surgery may be required to remove the string if it extends beyond the mouth. If a mouth infection has developed, antibiotics will be required to clear the bacteria.

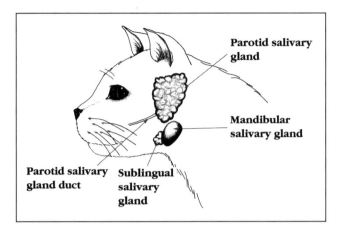

2-12 Salivary glands

DISORDERS OF THE SALIVARY GLANDS

The feline has four pairs of salivary glands, each with a different name. The pairs are the sublingual, mandibular, parotid and zygomatic (see figure 2-12). Their primary function is to produce saliva, which lubricates food and contains the enzyme ptyalin, which aids in digestion. Saliva production goes on constantly, with or without the presence of food. "Unused" saliva is simply swallowed.

EXCESSIVE DROOLING—PTYALISM

Excessive drooling may be caused by several conditions. There may be too much saliva production, the animal may not be swallowing or malformed lips may be letting saliva drain from the mouth. Unlike some dogs, normal cats do not drool excessively. Certain drugs, such as organophosphates occasionally used in flea preparations, may stimulate an overproduction of saliva. Newer and safer insecticides such as pyrethrins are not likely to cause this. Viral diseases such as rabies, tonsillitis and foreign bodies of the mouth may have excessive salivation as a symptom. The most common causes of drooling are infections of the mouth or gums.

What Are the Symptoms?
Saliva will form long filaments that hang or, in most cases, simply drip from the mouth.

What Are the Risks?
Drooling by itself is not harmful. The causes of drooling may have other, even fatal, implications. Diseases such as rabies may be fatal.

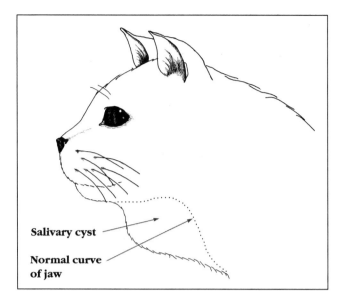

2-13   Salivary cyst

Drooling due to lip fold abnormalities can cause infections of the skin and areas that surround the mouth. The mouth should be examined closely for signs of gum or tooth disease.

What Is the Treatment?
The cause of drooling must be identified. Is the problem overproduction of saliva, an inability to swallow or simply the lip fold conformation? Were organophosphate drugs recently used to treat worms or fleas? Inability to swallow correctly always has an underlying medical problem that must be identified. For abnormal lip folds surgery can be performed to alter the lip structure and prevent further drooling. Always thoroughly examine the mouth for gum or tooth infections and foreign bodies of the mouth.

SIALOCELE (RANULA)

Occasionally, saliva will accumulate under the skin causing a large cyst structure. The cause is unknown, but most commonly it's due to injury. Damage to a salivary gland or duct may cause leakage of saliva under the skin.

What Are the Symptoms?
The most common salivary glands to be involved are the sublingual glands. They or their ducts can leak and cause saliva to accumulate under the chin or under the tongue (see figure 2-13).

What Are the Risks?

Salivary accumulations generally are not painful, and most patients have no other abnormalities.

What Is the Treatment?

A cure is usually achieved by removing the salivary gland that is producing the saliva. Specialized dye studies may need to be performed by a veterinarian to identify the involved gland. Removal of the glands has no long-term effects on the patient.

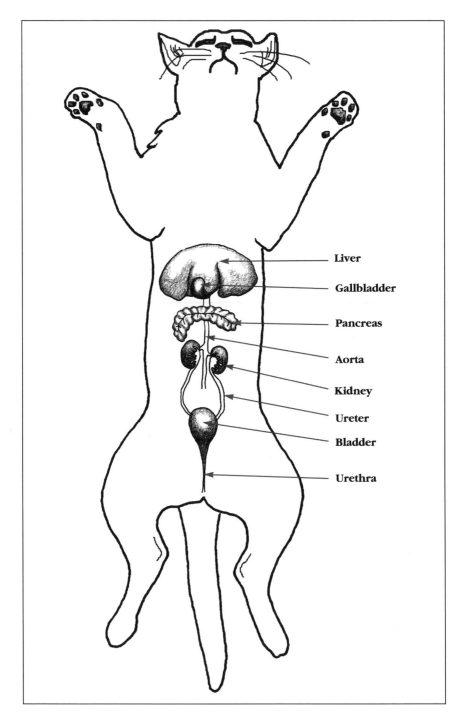

Liver

Gallbladder

Pancreas

Aorta

Kidney

Ureter

Bladder

Urethra

3-1 Digestive and other organs of the cat

CHAPTER 3

The Digestive Organs—
Liver, Pancreas and Gallbladder

For this chapter the digestive system will include only the following organs of digestion: the liver, pancreas and gallbladder. Disorders of the stomach and intestines are discussed in Chapter 4, "The Digestive Tract."

The **liver, gallbladder** and **pancreas** all provide substances to aid the digestion of food that takes place within the intestine (see figure 3-1).

The **liver** is the largest internal organ of the body (see figure 3-2) and has many functions. It stores sugar and vitamins and produces proteins and vitamins. It also filters wastes from the blood, digests fats and removes certain toxins, or poisons, from the body. Any disorder affecting the liver may cause a variety of signs or symptoms. *Bile* produced by the liver plays an important role in digestion. Bile is a waste product synthesized from the disintegration of old red blood cells. Bile functions aid digestion of fats consumed in the cat's diet. Bile produced by the liver is stored in a small balloon-like structure called the **gallbladder** (see figure 3-3). The gallbladder is connected to the **small intestine** by a tube called the **bile duct.** The bile duct carries bile to a section of the small intestine where it breaks down fats.

Bile acids are components of liver bile. Bile acids act like a detergent to convert fat globules into water-soluble nutrients. This allows the body to absorb them into the bloodstream through the intestinal wall. Bile also contains *bilirubin,* a pigment released from dead red blood cells that is responsible for the brown color of feces. If the liver becomes diseased, a frequently seen phenomena is jaundice (icterus). *Jaundice* is a buildup of pigments such as bilirubin in the bloodstream resulting in a yellowing of the skin, gums and whites of the eyes.

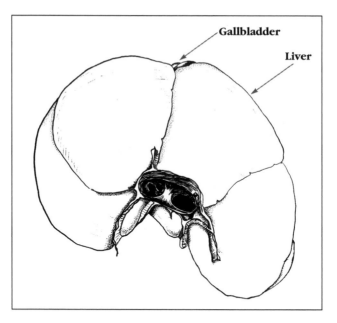

3-2   Liver

As described before, the **gallbladder** is a balloon-like structure located next to the liver. It stores and concentrates bile. Once the cat eats, the gallbladder is stimulated to deposit bile to the small intestine for fat digestion and excretion.

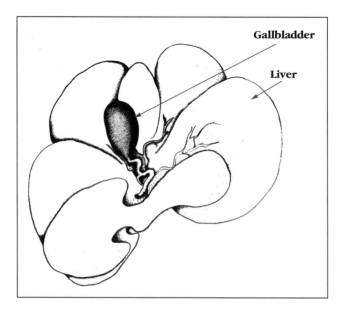

3-3   Gallbladder

Unlike the gallbladder, the **pancreas** is an organ that functions independently from the liver. The pancreas is a small ribbon-like structure located near, and attached to, the wall of the small intestine (see figure 3-4). The pancreas has two major functions; it produces insulin to aid in sugar absorption for the blood, and it produces important enzymes to aid in the digestion of proteins and lipids (fats). These enzymes travel from the pancreas to the small intestine through a small tube called the pancreatic duct.

Specifically, the pancreas produces two major protein digestive enzymes called *trypsin* and *chymotrypsin*. Fat digestion is aided by enzymes called lipases, which are also produced by the pancreas. Without these enzymes, cats would not be able to break down these important dietary constituents.

DISORDERS OF THE LIVER

Due to the liver's involvement in digestion, red blood cell metabolism, protein synthesis and other functions, diseases of the liver affect a wide range of the body's systems. Because the liver filters and detoxifies

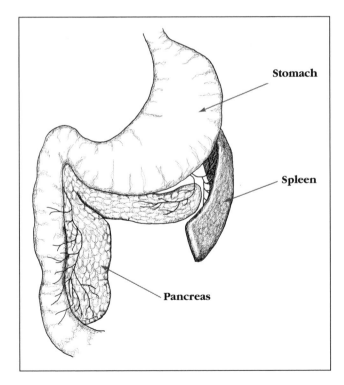

3-4 Pancreas

blood, it is very susceptible to toxins and infections. The fact that it is the largest internal organ also makes it susceptible to trauma. Because of the liver's many roles, disorders are frequently serious. Unlike other organs of the body, the *liver does have some capability to regenerate and replenish damaged cells.* Because of this, many disorders only temporarily affect the patient until the liver can recover.

FATTY LIVER DISEASE (HEPATIC LIPIDOSIS)

The liver is one of the main organs involved in the metabolism of fats. As with humans, some fat is actually stored in the cells of the cat's liver. In a normal cat, fat generally comprises a very small percentage of actual liver weight. Ninety-five percent of the liver is actually comprised of non-fat materials.

A cat with a fatty liver disorder, however, will have abnormally high fat deposits within the liver cells. Although the exact cause of excess fat storage within the liver is unknown, we do know that hormones that help to control fat metabolism may not be at the proper levels, and some patients may be diabetic, which alters fat metabolism. Despite the cause, if excess fat is stored within the liver cells, the fat-containing cells "crowd out" the normal cells thus preventing the liver from functioning normally.

What Are the Symptoms?
A cat with advanced fatty liver disease will have a failing liver. On initial observation, there is no way to diagnose this fatty infiltration. A liver biopsy provides the final diagnosis. As in other instances of liver failure, the patient may vomit, have diarrhea, lose weight and may appear icteric (jaundiced). Although most patients are overweight when the condition first develops, this is not always the case.

What Are the Risks?
A cat with fatty liver disease may be ill. In advanced stages the liver is unable to function and death may result. It is important to search for other underlying causes, such as diabetes mellitus (see Chapter 7). By correcting these disorders the chances of survival can be increased.

What Is the Treatment?
There is no specific treatment for a patient with fatty liver disease. If an underlying cause such as diabetes mellitus can be identified, it is crucial that it be treated immediately. Choline and methionine have been used as a therapy, but there is no scientific evidence to support their

benefits. Since choline and methionine are available in adequate levels in commercial cat foods, it is unlikely that supplementation has any positive effect on hepatic lipidosis.

LIVER TUMORS

Although not common, cancer of the liver is occasionally seen in cats. In most instances, cancer of the liver is the result of a cancerous spread from another area. Lymphosarcoma is the most commonly involved tumor of the liver. Lymphosarcoma isn't usually isolated to the liver, and tumors will be found elsewhere such as in the lungs, kidneys or lymph nodes.

What Are the Symptoms?
Most patients with liver cancer will show extreme weight loss coupled with jaundice, vomiting and/or diarrhea.

What Are the Risks?
Cancer of the liver is always serious and life threatening. If the tumor is malignant, as in lymphosarcoma, most patients survive only weeks to months.

What Is the Treatment?
Occasionally a cancer of the liver can be cured by early detection and a surgical removal of the affected areas. With lymphosarcoma, a complete recovery is rare and the disease is almost always fatal.

HEPATITIS

The term hepatitis describes an infection or inflammation of the liver. The cause may be viral, bacterial, parasitic or toxin-related. Well-known feline infectious diseases such as **f**eline **i**nfectious **p**eritonitis (FIP) may be the cause. Coal tar shampoo is an example of a product that is toxic to the liver of the cat.

What Are the Symptoms?
A cat with hepatitis will usually have a fever, vomit, diarrhea, weight loss and possibly be icteric (jaundice or yellow skin).

What Are the Risks?
Any disease of the liver is potentially serious. The liver plays a principal role in the body's metabolism. Serious infections may result in death.

What Is the Treatment?

Treatment of hepatitis is dependent on identifying the cause. Antibiotics frequently help if the cause is bacterial. If a toxin is suspected, the cat must be removed from the source. Some instances, such as those caused by **f**eline **i**nfectious **p**eritonitis (FIP), are not treatable. A vaccine is available to protect cats against FIP. For a more complete description of feline infectious peritonitis, please see Chapter 16, "Infectious Feline Diseases."

DISORDERS OF THE GALLBLADDER

As previously mentioned, the gallbladder is a small balloon-like structure connected to the liver. Its primary function is to store bile produced by the liver cells. The stored bile is then released by the gallbladder and travels via the bile duct to the small intestine where it aids in the digestive process.

GALL(BLADDER) STONES

As in humans, occasionally a feline patient will be diagnosed with gallstones. The fats making up bile may clump and become a solid mass referred to as a stone. The "stones" form within the gallbladder and can even pass into the ducts causing an obstruction in the normal bile flow.

What Are the Symptoms?

Most cats with gallstones show no symptoms whatsoever as these stones simply remain in the gallbladder. However, problems can arise if the stones become large or move into the bile duct and block the flow of bile from the liver or intestines. Patients with a blocked flow of bile may have a loose, clay-colored stool. In severe instances, jaundice may develop making the gums and skin take on a yellow appearance.

What Are the Risks?

Unless the flow of bile is interrupted, no risks are associated with gallstones. If bile flow is partially blocked, then bile may flow backwards into the liver causing a liver upset. A complete bile duct obstruction is serious, causing congestion and a decreased ability of the organ to function correctly. This has the same effect as any serious hepatitis.

What Is the Treatment?

Surgical removal of the gallstones to restore the normal flow of bile is the preferred treatment. It is not known why stones initially form, but surgical removal is very successful. Future stone formation is possible in cats prone to this disorder.

GALLBLADDER RUPTURE

Occasionally following a traumatic accident, such as a blow to the abdomen, the gallbladder may rupture. This allows the bile to spill directly into the abdomen and not reach the intestine.

What Are the Symptoms?
Initially there may be no noticeable symptoms. However, gallbladder contents, namely bile, are very caustic to other organs and the lining of the abdominal cavity. As bile leaks from the rupture, it irritates all exposed surfaces in the abdomen. Typical signs include fever and extreme abdominal pain as a peritonitis (inflammation of the abdominal cavity) is caused. Normal bile often contains bacteria from the liver and worsens the peritonitis.

What Are the Risks?
A ruptured gallbladder is life threatening. Peritonitis due to bile spill is a progressive disorder leading to severe inflammation, with adhesions forming between various abdominal structures.

What Is the Treatment?
Surgery is required to repair the rupture. If the damage is severe, the majority of the gallbladder can be removed with no serious consequences. Supportive care, anti-inflammatory drugs as well as antibiotics are used to treat the peritonitis.

DISORDERS OF THE PANCREAS

The pancreas is a small ribbon-like structure located in the abdomen near the stomach. It has many functions including aiding digestion and producing hormones, most notably insulin. Disorders of the pancreas are more common in the dog than in the cat, but nevertheless feline pancreatic disorders may occur.

PANCREATITIS

An inflammation of the pancreas is referred to as a pancreatitis. Although the cause is usually unknown, it may be caused by infection or trauma to the abdomen.

What Are the Symptoms?

Usually the cat has a painful, tender abdomen. Diarrhea and vomiting are usually present along with a loss of appetite. Frequently there is increased thirst, and there may be a fever.

What Are the Risks?

A disorder of the pancreas is serious, although not always life threatening. Immediate treatment should be sought to prevent a further decline in the cat's health caused by vomiting and diarrhea coupled with a loss of appetite.

What Is the Treatment?

Many patients respond well to the administration of antibiotics and steroids (cortisones). Although many cases are treatable, death may result. Steroids help relieve the inflammation while antibiotics fight bacteria if they are present.

DIABETES MELLITUS

Please see Chapter 7, "Hormone Disorders."

C H A P T E R   4

The Digestive Tract

The principal organs in the digestive tract are the **esophagus, stomach, small** and **large intestines, cecum** and **colon** (see figure 4-1). The digestive tract transports food from the mouth to the anus where it is eliminated from the body. As food moves through the intestinal tract, it is digested or broken down into nutrients that are absorbed through the intestinal walls. These nutrients are then transferred by the bloodstream to the tissues of the body to be used as fuel. Each portion of the digestive tract performs specialized tasks to aid in the transfer and digestion of food.

DISORDERS OF THE ESOPHAGUS

The esophagus is a small hose-like tube that leads from the mouth to the stomach. From the mouth, it follows a straight path through the neck and chest, where it passes near the heart, then through the diaphragm muscle and finally enters into the stomach. The esophagus walls are composed of muscles that move in wave-like contractions to push food into the stomach. It takes about five seconds for a cat's food to move from the mouth to the stomach. Surgery to the esophagus is always difficult because of the location within the chest and its poor rate of healing.

CONGENITAL MEGAESOPHAGUS

A megaesophagus occurs when the esophagus has lost its muscle tone. Rather than appearing like a muscular hose, it dilates into a thin, flaccid, "bag-like" tube (see figure 4-2). Most cases are congenital and are probably caused by an inadequate nerve function due to the improper development of the esophageal nerve supply.

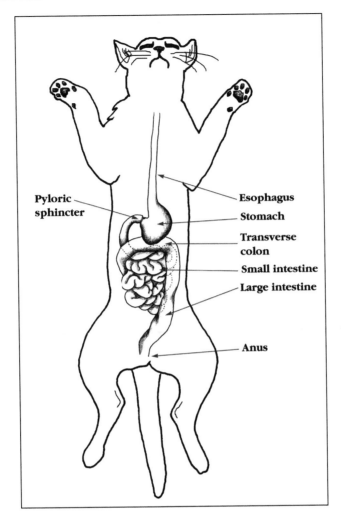

Pyloric sphincter

Esophagus

Stomach

Transverse colon

Small intestine

Large intestine

Anus

4-1   Digestive tract of the cat

What Are the Symptoms?

The patient tends to regurgitate or vomit food shortly after eating. The diseased esophagus lacks the muscular tone to move food to the stomach. Ingested food is swallowed, but sits within the esophagus until regurgitated back up. Some food, particularly liquids, may pass into the stomach.

What Are the Risks?

Usually, a megaesophagus is a permanent situation. Sometimes an infection or irritation of the nerve supply may cause temporary symptoms, but this is rare. Megaesophagus is generally a permanent condition that must be dealt with.

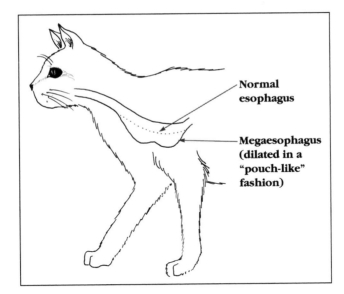

4-2   Congenital megaesophagus

What Is the Treatment?

Congenital megaesophagus has no known cure. Patients affected must be fed liquid diets. The food is usually placed in an elevated position so the patients eat while standing on the hind limbs. This elevated eating stance allows liquid food to use gravity to help get to the stomach. With these methods many patients can survive and do well.

NORMAL REGURGITATION

It is not uncommon for cats to regurgitate food that has never entered the stomach. The normal cat, especially those that ingest large amounts of hair, will occasionally regurgitate food. The authors generally do not consider one regurgitation episode or less per week as abnormal.

What Are the Symptoms?

A cat that regurgitates food will appear to have vomited. Vomit comes from the stomach however, and is usually accompanied by yellow, bile-stained stomach fluids. Regurgitated food is from the esophagus and usually appears simply as chewed food, usually in a linear mass, the shape of the esophagus. Hair may or may not be present.

What Are the Risks?

A cat that occasionally regurgitates is considered normal and not at risk. It is probably nature's way of helping to prevent hairballs, and perhaps, to some extent, overeating.

What Is the Treatment?

Because an occasional regurgitation is considered normal, there is no treatment. However it is important for the owner to note if the regurgitative episodes are becoming more frequent. If they are, a veterinary exam should be performed.

FOREIGN BODIES IN THE ESOPHAGUS

The esophagus, being a tube-like structure, is capable of a certain amount of dilation to allow larger pieces of food to reach the stomach. Occasionally felines ingest objects other than normal food, and a common place for this foreign material to lodge is in the esophagus. Objects typically lodge near the heart as this is where the esophagus is unable to expand to its widest point. Balls, rocks, sticks, coins, yarn and poultry bones are all examples of foreign bodies that may lodge in this area.

What Are the Symptoms?

Once the esophagus is blocked in this manner, food usually is regurgitated within a few minutes after eating.

What Are the Risks?

A foreign body in the esophagus is always serious. Sharp objects can puncture or wear away the esophageal muscle wall, allowing food and bacteria to enter the chest cavity. A severe and *life-threatening pneumonia can develop.*

What Is the Treatment?

Treatment is aimed at removing the object. This may be accomplished by anesthetizing the patient and removing the object via the mouth or pushing it on and into the stomach. In many instances the chest cavity and esophagus must be surgically opened and the object removed. Although this type of surgery poses a great risk to the patient, the final outcome can be excellent.

DISORDERS OF THE STOMACH

The feline stomach is like a sac designed to store large volumes of food and begin the digestive process (see figure 4-3). The storage of ingested food is short term, and once eaten, most food will leave the stomach within 12 hours. The esophagus carries food to the stomach. At the base of the esophagus where it enters the stomach there is a small valve-like structure called the **cardiac sphincter.** Food exits the stomach into the first part of the small intestine called the **duodenum.** A small muscular valve called the **pyloric sphincter** separates the stomach from the duodenum. On the interior surface of the stomach are a series of folds called gastric folds (see figure 4-4). These folds function to help grind and digest food. The inner stomach lining secretes acids and enzymes to break down food as the initial step in the digestive process. Once the initial stomach digestive process is complete, the partially digested food leaves the stomach through the pyloric sphincter area and then enters the duodenum, the first portion of the small intestine.

GASTRIC ULCERS

Ulcers are small, pitted areas that develop when the inner intestinal lining is worn away (see figure 4-5). As in humans, stress or a "nervous" stomach can cause ulcers. This is probably due to the higher-than-normal levels of stomach acids produced in the nervous patient. The stomach cells secrete these acids, and excess levels can irritate and erode the stomach lining. Certain anti-inflammatory drugs such as aspirin, phenylbutazone, ibuprofen and cortisones can also lead to stomach ulcers, especially if used in high quantities or for long

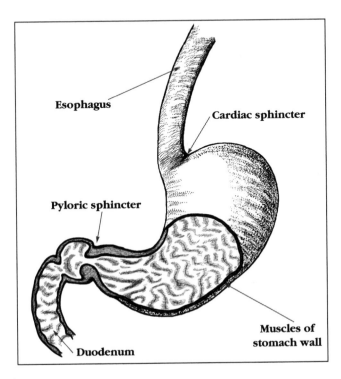

Esophagus

Cardiac sphincter

Pyloric sphincter

Muscles of stomach wall

Duodenum

4-3 Stomach

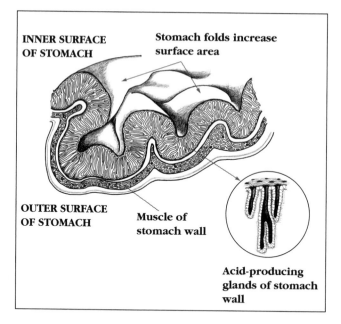

INNER SURFACE
OF STOMACH

Stomach folds increase
surface area

OUTER SURFACE
OF STOMACH

Muscle of
stomach wall

Acid-producing
glands of stomach
wall

4-4   Stomach detail

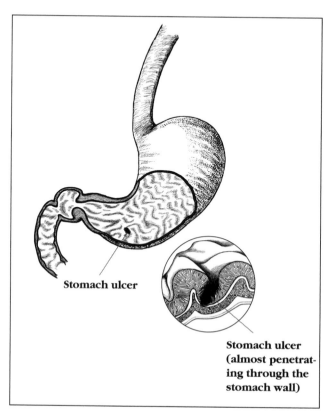

Stomach ulcer

Stomach ulcer
(almost penetrat-
ing through the
stomach wall)

4-5   Stomach ulcer

periods of time. Bacteria may also colonize the stomach lining and cause ulcerations.

What Are the Symptoms?

Gastric ulcerations range from moderate to severe. Typical signs include vomiting, occasionally with blood, and a poor appetite. If the ulcers are pitted deep into the stomach tissues, severe hemorrhaging may occur, leading to anemia and black, tar-like stools. The stools appear dark as a result of blood becoming partially digested through the small intestine and colon.

What Are the Risks?

Most patients tolerate gastric ulcers very well. In fact, many moderate ulcers heal on their own and even if they persist, cause nothing more than an occasional stomach upset. Severe ulcerations, however, can lead to death due to excessive blood loss and/or complete perforation of the stomach wall.

What Is the Treatment?

A careful evaluation of the pet's history is important. Any potential ulcer-causing drugs should be discontinued in this patient. Drug therapy is beneficial. Antacids such as Digel can be used to help counteract the excess acid production. As in humans, various other drugs such as cimetidine (Tagamet) are available to help decrease the stomach acid production. Coating agents such as Kaopectate or Pepto Bismol are also beneficial. Antibiotics are helpful if bacteria are present.

PYLORIC STENOSIS

Where the stomach empties into the duodenum, there is a circular, valve-like structure of muscle called the pyloric sphincter. The pyloric sphincter constricts and dilates, regulating the flow of food from the stomach into the small intestine. Occasionally, for unknown reasons, the pyloric sphincter abnormally constricts or spasms, causing a narrowing (stenosis) of the entrance into the small intestine. Nervous individuals seem to develop this condition more frequently than others.

What Are the Symptoms?

Intermittent vomiting within one to two hours of eating is the most common sign. The food will appear undigested, looking much as it did when first eaten. The sphincter may not always be constricting or spastic, therefore some meals may pass without being regurgitated. Additionally, water and liquid diets will pass through the narrowed sphincter easier than bulk-type foods. In severe cases, the cat may lose weight.

What Are the Risks?

Many patients live normal lives with only occasional episodes of vomiting. It appears the muscular spasms are not always constant in these cases. If a patient is exhibiting severe stomach outflow restrictions from a more constant pyloric stenosis, then severe weight loss and even death can result.

What Is the Treatment?

A diagnosis is not always easy. A careful history of vomiting in relation to eating must be evaluated. Barium studies with radiographs (X-rays) may reveal the narrowed stomach outflow. Once diagnosed, surgery provides the best cure. The pyloric sphincter, being a narrow muscular band, can be surgically severed, thus eliminating the constricting efforts. Additionally, the stomach outflow area can be surgically widened, allowing food to pass into the duodenum. The outcome after surgery is excellent.

FOREIGN BODIES IN THE STOMACH

Felines by nature tend to ingest objects other than normal food. Any material found within the stomach other than food or water is termed a foreign body. The authors have found many items within the stomach of cats, including coins, yarn, buttons, small balls, paper clips, rocks, hairballs, Easter basket grass, nails, tinsel, fish hooks and other small objects. (see figure 4-6).

What Are the Symptoms?

A patient with a foreign body in the stomach will almost always vomit, often repeatedly and violently. If the object is small, such as a paper clip, the vomiting may only be occasional. Frequently the vomiting occurs shortly after eating. The vomitus will usually contain only the last meal ingested. The food will appear undigested or very similar to the way it did before eating. Some cats with a foreign body in their stomach will stop eating any food.

What Are the Risks?

Small foreign bodies such as a coin or a button may eventually pass completely through the stomach and intestinal tract and be eliminated from the body in the feces. Larger foreign bodies may remain in the stomach for a long period of time and cause severe damage to the stomach. Left untreated, these instances become serious and end in death.

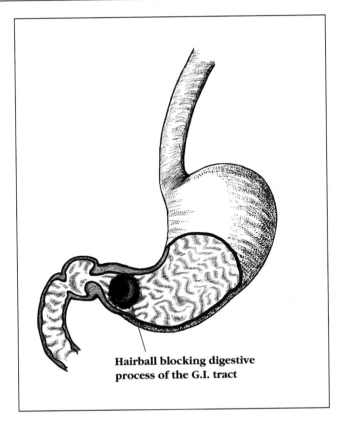

Hairball blocking digestive
process of the G.I. tract

4-6   Foreign body in stomach (hairball)

What Is the Treatment?

The ingestion of small objects may require no treatment. The patient is closely monitored for vomiting until the object passes from the body in the feces. It may take one to four days for the object to pass. The diagnosis of a foreign body can usually be confirmed with radiographs (X-rays) and occasionally the simple palpitation of the stomach area. Surgery is required to remove objects that are too large to pass from the body naturally. To prevent hairballs, a feeding of a feline hairball remedy twice weekly is recommended. This helps lubricate the hair and allows it to pass harmlessly through the digestive tract.

GASTRITIS

A gastritis is used to describe an inflammation or infection of the stomach. As in humans, viruses and bacteria can irritate the stomach and cause a gastritis. Additionally, the ingestion of spoiled foodstuffs such as soured milk can irritate the stomach lining.

What Are the Symptoms?

A patient with a gastritis will generally vomit, refuse to eat and be lethargic. Frequently, the temperature is elevated above the normal 101.5 degrees Fahrenheit. If a virus or bacteria is involved, the gastritis may eventually progress to involve the intestines as well, causing diarrhea.

What Are the Risks?

Most instances of gastritis are not serious. However, if the vomiting becomes severe or the signs persist for more than 24 hours, veterinary attention should be sought.

What Is the Treatment?

A patient with a mild upset stomach can benefit from gastric soothing or coating preparations such as Pepto Bismol. Generally, it is best to withhold food, but not water. Withholding food will allow the stomach to rest. Bland diets can be offered once the stomach has settled. Water should be given in small amounts frequently rather than allowing the animal to drink as much as it wants at one time. If the vomiting persists, diarrhea develops, or the body temperature is excessively high (greater than 103 degrees Fahrenheit), veterinary attention should be sought. A veterinarian will check the patient for dehydration due to lack of fluid intake and fluid lost in diarrhea or vomitus. Intravenous fluids can be used to replace lost fluids. Antibiotics that kill bacteria are used if necessary. Various medications are available to decrease vomiting.

TUMORS OF THE STOMACH

Although not common, stomach cancer occasionally develops in the feline. The main type of cancer involving the stomach is a malignant tumor called an adenocarcinoma. This type of tumor arises from the glandular cells of the stomach lining.

What Are the Symptoms?

A patient with stomach cancer generally loses weight, vomits and fails to eat. Blood may or may not be present in the vomit. The vomiting may initially be infrequent, increasing with time.

What Are the Risks?

Cancer of the stomach is always serious. Even with treatment the long-term prognosis is poor. Most cases are in the advanced stage before a proper diagnosis can be confirmed. Adenocarcinomas frequently spread to other areas of the body, making treatment even more difficult.

What Is the Treatment?

Surgical removal of the cancerous stomach areas are performed. Occasionally, large portions of the stomach wall are diseased and must be removed. Adenocarcinomas of the stomach may spread to other organs such as the liver and the lymph nodes. Tumors at these sites must also be isolated and removed. The long-term success of treatment is generally poor.

DISORDERS OF THE SMALL INTESTINE

The small intestine is a tube-like structure that extends between the stomach and large intestine. It is the longest portion of the intestinal tract. The small intestine of the feline has three parts. The first portion, which attaches to the stomach, is named the duodenum. The middle and longest portion is called the jejunum. The shortest part, which is connected to the large intestine, is called the ileum.

The duodenum attaches to the stomach and is relatively short. It does, however, have very important functions. The gallbladder and pancreas connect to the duodenum by the bile and pancreatic ducts respectively. Digestive enzymes and secretions are produced by the liver and pancreas, pass through these ducts and then mix with food in the duodenum.

The longest area of the small intestine, the jejunum, is rich in small finger-like projections called villi. Villi protrude inward into the food contents and provide a surface to absorb nutrients. Intestinal contents of the jejunum empty into the ileum and from there pass into the colon.

Diseases of the small intestine are usually not confined to just one area and therefore are simply discussed as small intestinal disorders.

SMALL INTESTINAL INFECTIONS—INFECTIOUS ENTERITIS

An enteritis is a term used to describe an inflammation or infection of the small intestine. In the feline many bacteria and viruses have been implicated as a cause of enteritis. Among them are salmonellosis, feline panleukopenia, feline leukemia virus (FeLV) (see Chapter 16) and others. Most of these organisms affect other areas of the body as well; however, some of their primary signs are associated with their intestinal effects.

What Are the Symptoms?

Diarrhea is the most common sign associated with a diseased small intestine. With an enteritis, the temperature is commonly elevated. However, this is not always the case—especially when viruses are concerned. A characteristic fetid odor is detected from the feces. The diarrhea may be green and profuse, almost like pea soup. If the intestinal wall is damaged due to the infection, there may also be blood in the stool. If the blood is from the first portion of the small intestine (duodenum) it will be digested and appear black or tar-like. If the bleeding is occurring near the colon, it may appear red.

What Are the Risks?

Any patient with an intestinal infection is severely ill. Depending on the cause, the recovery period may be days to weeks. Occasionally patients will die, especially if less than six months of age, although all ages are vulnerable. The death rate is higher in the young and the geriatric. Most organisms are highly contagious and an outbreak may involve many animals in the household and vicinity at one time.

What Is the Treatment?

A mild bout of infectious enteritis may require no treatment. The patient may have only a mild diarrhea for one or two days then spontaneously recover. In more severe instances, the patient will need medication as an aid in stopping or controlling the diarrhea. Nutrients and fluids may need to be administered intravenously or subcutaneously until the patient recovers. Antibiotics are helpful if the causative agent is a bacteria. Antibiotics also help prevent bacteria from secondarily complicating viral diseases. Kaopectate and other intestinal coating agents are beneficial in mild cases. In some cases medication that slows down the secretions of the intestinal tract can also be administered. The exact treatment varies by age, cause and severity. Patients should be monitored closely.

HERNIAS AND BOWEL STRANGULATIONS

Some cats have abnormal openings through the muscular abdominal wall. Abdominal contents, such as sections of the intestine, masses of fat, other organs, etc. may pass through these tear-like openings called hernias. Hernias typically occur at one or more sites. Umbilical hernias tend to occur in young cats as a result of weakness or lack of normal closure where the umbilical cord passed through the abdominal wall. This is the navel or "belly button" (see figure 4-7).

The other common hernia location is in the inguinal area on both sides of the abdomen where the rear legs join the body. This area is more commonly affected in males. As in humans, this area on both sides of the penis has openings that allow the testicles to descend from the abdomen into the scrotum. These natural openings through the abdominal muscles are called the inguinal rings. Occasionally the inguinal rings are too large, or they tear, allowing a larger opening,

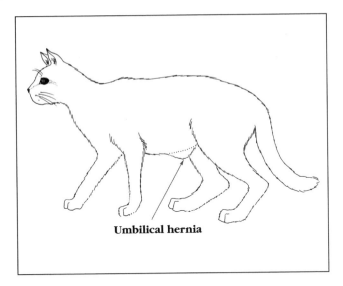

Umbilical hernia

4-7 Umbilical hernia

which permits a hernia to occur. One or both sides may be affected. Hernias are nothing more than abnormal openings through the muscles of the abdomen through which the abdominal contents pass. Skin still covers the area. Inguinal hernias generally occur later in life and, as in humans, are commonly the result of stress on the abdominal muscles, such as trauma.

What Are the Symptoms?
The most commonly noted symptom is a bulge of the belly skin at the hernia site. This bulge is due to tissues protruding from inside the abdomen and pushing outward on the skin. In the case of umbilical hernias, the bulge will occur directly over the navel. Inguinal hernias will be noted as a bulge next to the penis. Inguinal hernias may affect one or both sides simultaneously.

What Are the Risks?
Hernias, openings through the muscles, are not painful and cause no discomfort. The risk they pose is one of organ strangulation. A piece of intestine or even the bladder may pass through the muscle opening and become constricted. The constriction can cut off the blood supply to the organ and result in tissue death (see figure 4-8). Left untreated, this will lead to death. Oddly enough, large hernias pose less risk than small ones. This is because they are less likely than a small hernia to strangulate the organ. Large hernias restrict the blood supply less than small openings. In some instances, a very young kitten (less than six weeks of age) will have a small umbilical hernia that will heal shut or

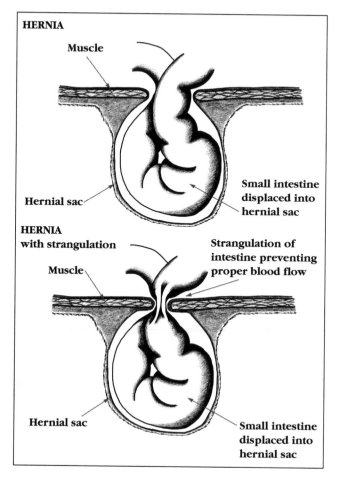

4-8 Hernia schematic

"scar over." In general, a hernia in any animal over four months of age should be corrected to prevent possible organ strangulation.

What Is the Treatment?

As with humans, treatment involves surgery. A veterinarian can surgically open the skin and close the abnormal opening that extends through the abdominal muscles. A full recovery is expected.

FOREIGN BODIES IN THE SMALL INTESTINE

Cats occasionally ingest objects that are indigestible and not intended as food. These are termed foreign bodies. Examples include sticks, weeds, coins, hairballs, marbles and strings. Although all of these objects may pass harmlessly through the entire digestive tract and exit

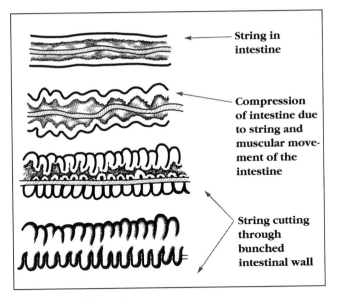

4-9   Foreign body in small intestine

in the stool, they can become lodged within the stomach and/or intestines. When foreign bodies cannot pass through to the feces, they may cause a complete or partial intestinal blockage. In the cat, the most severe cases we have seen were caused by string, yarn or fish line. Because of their length, these are termed linear foreign bodies.

Linear foreign bodies are especially dangerous as they commonly involve several areas of the gastrointestinal tract. An 18-inch piece of yarn, for instance, may wrap around the tongue with portions being swallowed passing through the esophagus, stomach and small intestine. As the normal intestinal muscular contractions occur, they pull and tighten the intestine over the string much like an accordion (see figure 4-9). As the string tries to pass, it tightens and may cut through the tongue, esophagus, stomach and intestines, causing severe and life-threatening damage. Intestinal contents may leak through the damaged areas into the abdominal cavity and cause a peritonitis. If the string passes entirely to the small intestine, it may affect only that area.

What Are the Symptoms?
A foreign body in the intestinal tract will usually cause the patient to stop eating and drinking. If the intestines are obstructed, severe vomiting may develop, usually with little or no stool being produced. Dehydration will follow. Blood may appear in the feces if the foreign body has irritated but not blocked the intestines. As with all foreign bodies, if they become lodged, the patient usually is very ill within one week. If damage is done to the intestinal tract a fever may be present.

What Are the Risks?

All foreign bodies of the intestinal tract can become serious and life threatening. *Linear foreign bodies and those causing complete obstruction will usually cause death within seven days if left untreated.*

What Is the Treatment?

Once the diagnosis of a gastrointestinal foreign body is made, the offending object(s) must be surgically removed *at once*. Linear foreign bodies such as string pose the greatest risk as the intestinal tract may need to be surgically entered in several locations to repair it in sections. Occasionally entire portions of the intestines are damaged beyond repair and will need to be removed. There is really no way to prevent the ingestion of foreign bodies other than to limit the cat's access to such objects. Hairball remedies that are actually intestinal lubricants will help prevent the buildup of hairballs by helping the hair pass through the body in the stool. All cats that groom extensively or are prone to developing hairballs should be fed a hairball remedy on a regular basis.

PARASITIC ENTERITIS

Cats of all ages have the function of the small intestine compromised by parasites. Roundworms, tapeworms and hookworms are all found within the bowel of felines. Hookworms are the most devastating, as they attach to the intestinal wall, suck blood from the victim and damage the absorption surfaces of the intestine. All these worms are found within the small intestine; however, whipworms are generally located at the very end by the cecum and colon.

Although all ages of felines may become infested with parasites, the young are the most susceptible. Kittens are frequently born with (or acquire shortly after birth) parasites from their mother. Roundworms and hookworms are common in infants as they pass through the placenta or through the mother's milk. Tapeworms generally do not transfer directly from animal to animal. Fleas, fish, snails, rodents, rabbits and other insects serve as carriers of tapeworms. Once a pet ingests a carrier, the tapeworm will complete its life cycle. Fleas serve as the principal tapeworm reservoir for the feline.

What Are the Symptoms?

Many patients with intestinal parasites exhibit few or no symptoms. Routine fecal exams by a veterinarian will detect the parasites or their eggs, if present. Tapeworm segments occasionally are seen crawling about the anus of cats or on fresh stool. They resemble a piece of rice. Roundworms are spaghetti-like and may appear in the stool.

Diarrhea with or without blood, bloated abdomens and poor hair coats all indicate parasites.

What Are the Risks?

Mild parasitic infestations cause little harm to the pet. Roundworms and tapeworms are not blood suckers and do not damage the gut wall. They survive stomach acids and bathe in the digesting food, competing with the pet for nutrients.

Hookworms are more serious in that they suck blood and destroy areas of the gut wall when feeding. Severe infestations can cause blood loss leading to anemia and death. A pet with parasites is not a healthy pet and should be treated at once.

What Is the Treatment?

A fecal exam by a veterinarian will help identify the types of parasites present. Each individual patient should have a routine fecal exam at least twice yearly. Various worming medications are available to kill the identified parasites. All kittens should be routinely wormed beginning at two or three weeks of age. Effective and safe wormers are readily available.

For a more complete discussion of these and other parasites, please refer to Chapter 15, "Common Feline Parasites."

TUMORS OF THE SMALL INTESTINE

As with other organs in the abdomen, the small intestine can occasionally become cancerous. The small intestine, being rich in glandular tissue, is particularly susceptible to tumors arising from those cells. These types of tumors are termed adenocarcinomas.

What Are the Symptoms?

The tumors can interrupt digestion and absorption, or lead to an intestinal blockage. Additionally, they often spread to the liver or lungs, affecting the normal function of these organs. The symptoms of intestinal cancer are varied, but can include weight loss, vomiting, diarrhea and anemia.

What Are the Risks?

All cases of intestinal cancer are serious and should be treated at once. Even with treatment, the long-term outcome is typically poor.

What Is the Treatment?

The affected areas are generally surgically removed and biopsied. Chemotherapy is occasionally used in conjunction with surgery. Therapy must be evaluated on an individual basis.

DISORDERS OF THE LARGE INTESTINE

The cat's large intestine basically connects the small intestine to the anus. Its primary function is to absorb water from feces as needed, thus maintaining the hydration level of the body. Its other function is to store fecal matter awaiting passage from the body.

The large intestine has several distinct parts. The **cecum** is a small, finger-like projection near the junction with the small intestine. Its function is unknown. The **colon** is the longest portion of the large intestine and terminates just inside the **anus** to the final portion called the **rectum.** The terms colon and large intestine are used interchangeably.

COLITIS

Colitis describes an inflammation of the colon. Although, the cause may be bacteria, stress, parasites and so on, there is often no detectable reason for the inflammation.

What Are the Symptoms?
Most patients with a colitis look and feel normal. They simply have loose stools, frequently with mucous and occasional flecks of blood. In severe cases, vomiting may occur. Due to pain associated with inflammation of the colon, some patients will experience severe pain when defecating and may actually try and stop the defecation process, thereby resulting in constipation. There may be constipation or diarrhea, but invariably there will be an abnormal defecation process. Diarrhea or a loose stool is more commonly encountered than is constipation.

What Are the Risks?
Most patients have no serious health risk. In cases when deep ulceration of the colon develops, the situation is more serious. Parasites should be eliminated if they are the suspected cause. Cats chronically affected may lose weight.

What Is the Treatment?
A rectal exam coupled with a colon wall biopsy will generally confirm a diagnosis. Fecal exams for colon parasites such as giardia should be performed in all cases of colitis. Bland diets will help the colon rest and heal. Antibiotics will help control bacteria causing colitis. Metronidazole (Flagyl) is commonly used in the treatment of colitis in the feline.

CONSTIPATION

Straining to defecate without passing the appropriate amount of stool is called constipation. The stool within the bowel is hard and unable to pass easily through the colon and out of the anus. Constipation can be the result of several factors. The most common cause of constipation is eating abnormal substances such as bones, sand, wood and other objects. Although readily eaten, objects such as chicken bones form hard, rock-like clumps of stool within the colon. Lack of water may also cause extra-hard stools. Some cases of constipation are from injuries to the colon where the damaged area may affect the cat's ability to defecate. A condition called megacolon (see below) may develop and be the cause of constipation. Long-haired breeds may develop hair mats covering the anal opening, preventing defecation. Rectal polyps and cancers, although not common, may contribute.

What Are the Symptoms?
Straining with little or no defecation is a common sign of constipation. Some liquid feces may pass, but the fecal mass is retained. The patient may lick or bite at its rear end as if something is wrong. In chronic cases there may be a reluctance to eat, or even vomiting.

What Are the Risks?
Simple constipation as a result of abnormally hard stool is usually not serious. To determine the exact risk, it is important to isolate the cause. Fortunately, 90 percent of all cases of constipation have no detectable causes and are simply diet related.

What Is the Treatment?
The patient should be examined to determine the cause. Is the stool simply too hard, or has the patient suffered an injury? Enemas may relieve the constipation. If a patient periodically encounters constipation, try changing foods. Avoid meat-only diets. Mineral oil and milk have laxative effects and are beneficial in some patients. Diets high in fiber are best in geriatric patients or those prone to chronic constipation. Unless the cat is in great discomfort, do not worry if a patient goes one or two days without passing a stool. Most instances of constipation will resolve themselves naturally within 48 hours. If more than 48 hours pass with no bowel movement, a veterinary exam is suggested.

MEGACOLON

Megacolon is a term used to describe a colon that is abnormally large in diameter (see figure 4-10). There are two forms of megacolon:

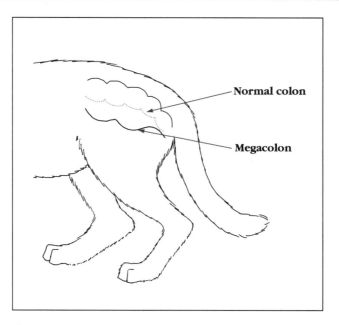

4-10   Megacolon

congenital and *acquired*. In the congenital form, the kitten is born with an abnormal nerve supply to the colon, which causes its muscles to be loose and flaccid.

Without proper innervation and therefore muscular tone, the colon dilates into a large, flaccid tube with a decreased ability to constrict and move food towards the anus.

Acquired megacolon develops in middle-aged and older cats. It is not known why the colon loses muscular tone, but it may be a result of the degeneration of a once-normal nerve supply. Repeated episodes of severe constipation may also damage the colon walls and lead to an acquired megacolon. Trauma such as a back injury may also damage the nerves supplying the colon. Regardless of cause, whether the megacolon is congenital or acquired, the end result is a dilated colon with poor muscle tone.

What Are the Symptoms?

With megacolon, the colon has poor or absent muscle tone. This leads to the inability to move feces to the anus for elimination from the body (defecation). This patient will become constipated and spend an abnormal length of time attempting to pass the stool. The difficulty in defecating will usually progress slowly, especially if the megacolon is acquired. If severe constipation develops, the patient may vomit and become dehydrated and anorexic.

What Are the Risks?

Megacolon is serious in that there is usually no way to correct the colon dysfunction. Commonly, the colon function will worsen over a period of months to years, occasionally to the point of no colonic mobility whatsoever. This patient will experience difficulty in defecation and in advanced cases may be totally unable to defecate.

What Is the Treatment?

It is not common to identify a treatable cause of megacolon. Occasionally a spinal injury may heal over time, in which case the colonic function may return. Ninety-five percent of all instances of megacolon, however, have no identifiable cause or specific treatment.

Warm water enemas will help alleviate constipation. The use of stool softeners and increasing the dietary fiber will help patients develop a softer, more easily passed stool. With megacolon, treatment is primarily aimed at managing the condition rather than attempting a total cure.

Surgical removal of the colon (colonectomy) is possible, but oftentimes the outcome is not favorable. In this procedure, the colon is removed and the small intestine is reattached to the rectum.

C H A P T E R 5

The Respiratory System

The respiratory system is basically comprised of the **nares** or **pharynx openings** into the nose, **sinuses** within the skull, **larynx, trachea** (windpipe), **bronchi** (the branch of the trachea going into the lungs) and the **lungs** (see figure 5-1).

The respiratory system functions as a mechanism for exchange. It removes carbon dioxide from the body and replaces it with oxygen. The feline's respiratory system also serves as a unique cooling system. Cats don't have sweat glands, so they can't perspire. To lower their body temperature they must breathe faster or pant. By breathing faster, warm air is exchanged from the body for the cooler outside air. Additionally, moisture within the respiratory system evaporates, further cooling these surfaces. The lungs' dual function is to exchange carbon dioxide for oxygen and to cool the body.

The act of breathing is relatively simple and is accomplished by the actions of the rib muscles (intercostal) and the movement of a large internal muscle called the **diaphragm.** The diaphragm muscle separates the chest, which contains the heart and lungs, from the abdomen, which holds the intestines, stomach, liver and bladder. As this great muscle moves toward the abdomen, it pulls fresh air and oxygen into the lungs. This is inhalation. The chest cavity surrounding the lungs is a vacuum that allows the lungs to inflate easily when the cat is breathing in. When the muscle moves forward away from the abdomen, it causes the lungs to compress and the body exhales old, used air.

As a cat inhales, fresh air moves through the nose or mouth, into the pharynx and larynx to the trachea. This rigid tube carries air to the bronchi that in turn supply oxygen to the lungs. A feline has one right and one left lung. The lungs are divided into sections or lobes. At the cellular level, the lungs are rich in air pockets called *alveoli*. It is in the alveoli that the blood makes contact with the individual cells of the lungs and oxygen is exchanged for carbon dioxide. Alveoli are

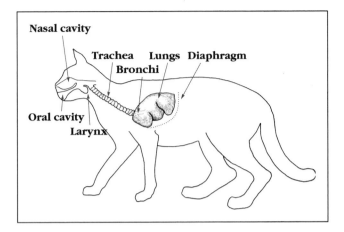

5-1 Respiratory system

supplied by a vast network of microscopic blood vessels known as capillaries, which allow the carbon dioxide to follow the opposite path; they pass into the bronchi, then the trachea through the larynx and pharynx, and finally exit through the nose or mouth.

In this section we will describe common disorders that affect the various components of the respiratory system.

THE NOSE

The nose is one entrance into the respiratory system (see figure 5-2). The nose is lined with folds of mucous membranes that clean and add moisture to the incoming air. The membrane surfaces are covered by mucous produced by cells throughout the respiratory system. Dirt and debris are caught within this mucous. The respiratory surfaces are also covered by small, hair-like structures called cilia. The cilia beat in a coordinated fashion to keep the mucous moving and they also filter and trap dust particles. As air swirls about the folds, particles such as pollen and dust are removed by the sticky mucous and cilia. This filters the air before it enters the more fragile lungs.

Cold air is warmed by the nose as well as the open spaces called sinuses, which form part of the nasal passages (see figure 5-3). Air moves in through the nasal opening, then through the nose and sinuses where it is cleansed and warmed. It then passes on through the pharynx to the opening in the trachea called the larynx. The nose also functions as an organ of smell. Any disorders affecting the nose may impede the cat's ability to smell. The cat does not, however, normally possess a keen sense of smell. The cat's olfactory lobes of the brain that detect odors are not as developed as those in many animals, including dogs. Cats detect food primarily by vision and not by smell. This probably accounts for a relatively poor sense of smell.

RHINITIS

An infection of the passages within the nose and nares is termed rhinitis. Cats are particularly susceptible to this condition, probably caused by short and relatively narrow nasal passages (nares). Cats with short (brachycephalic) faces, such as Persians, are the most affected, as their airways are even more constricted. Bacteria such as *Chlamydia* and *Staphylococcus* are common pathogens of the nose. Fungi and viruses may also cause nasal infections.

What Are the Symptoms?

Symptoms depend somewhat on the type of infection causing the disorder. In general, one may notice excessive nasal discharge, which may develop into a thick yellow or greenish mucous. The patient may sneeze frequently in attempts to clear the nasal passages of mucous. In advanced cases, the mucous may become bloody. This patient usually has difficulty smelling.

The nose may be hot *or* cold. The folk advice about a cold nose is not a good indicator of a cat's sickness or health. Normal patients may have hot, cold, dry or wet noses. The body temperature, however, is an important indicator. A patient with severe rhinitis may have an elevated body temperature. If this is the case, the patient generally becomes lethargic with a poor appetite.

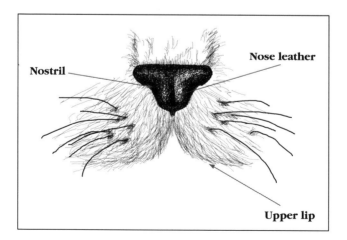

5-2 Nose

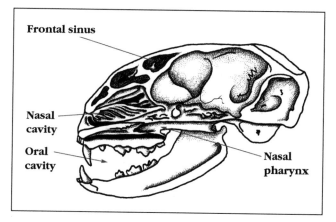

5-3 Nasal cavity

What Are the Risks?

This again depends on the exact organism(s) involved. Most cases remain confined to the nose and its sinuses and in these instances the risks are minimal. If, however, the infection(s) spread to the more delicate regions of the respiratory system such as the trachea, bronchi or lungs, then the patient may be affected more severely.

What Is the Treatment?

Any patient suffering from a nasal infection should rest and be isolated from other pets to minimize the spread of contagious diseases. If the symptoms persist or a fever develops, the patient should be examined *at once* by a veterinarian.

In chronic cases needing treatment, a veterinarian will usually perform a culture of the nasal mucous. This aids in identifying which organism(s) is responsible for the infection. Once this is performed, the appropriate medications are selected. Antihistamines such as Benadryl are occasionally used to help dry and open the airways. Antibiotics such as Amoxicillin, Tribrissen and Keflex are commonly used against bacterial infections. Vaporizers—the same ones used for humans—are also beneficial. Simply place the pet in a wire cage in a small area such as a bathroom, and vaporize the air. This moist air makes breathing easier.

NASAL FOREIGN BODY

Since the nose has openings, it is not uncommon for material other than air to enter its passages. Foreign material, usually called foreign bodies, may include hair, sticks, weeds, feathers and so on.

What Are the Symptoms?

The initial sign of having an object lodged within the nose is usually sneezing. The sneezing may range from mild to extremely violent. Bleeding may or may not occur. A nasal infection may develop if the foreign body is not removed. The infection is usually limited to the affected side only. This is important in distinguishing a typical nasal infection from a problem induced by a foreign body.

What Are the Risks?

Foreign bodies within the nasal passages are always serious. They can cause severe irritation and impede the patient's ability to breathe.

What Is the Treatment?

If possible, remove the foreign object at once with your fingers or tweezers. If the material is deeply embedded, seek veterinary assistance at once. Sedation or anesthesia may be necessary as many patients do not tolerate nasal examinations. Once the foreign body is removed, sneezing and bleeding usually stop and the airway heals.

THE LARYNX

The larynx is a circular organ composed of cartilage and muscle located at the entrance of the trachea (see figure 5-4). It is commonly known as the **Adam's apple.** The larynx houses the **vocal cords.** These small muscle bands create sounds, such as meowing, by vibrating. The larynx's other function is to close, thereby preventing food from entering the trachea when a cat swallows. It does this by closing a small flap of muscle over the laryngeal opening. This muscular flap is called the **epiglottis.**

Larynxes sometimes develop infections.

LARYNGITIS

Laryngitis is the term used to describe an infection or irritation of the larynx. Many conditions caused by viruses or bacteria such as strep throat, can also involve the larynx of the feline.

What Are the Symptoms?

Generally, a patient suffering with laryngitis will have an altered voice. In the cases of felines, one may notice a complete inability to vocalize. If the larynx swells, it can actually block air flow to the trachea, which causes the patient to have difficulty breathing. Laryngitis can be very painful; some patients will not eat to avoid having to swallow. There

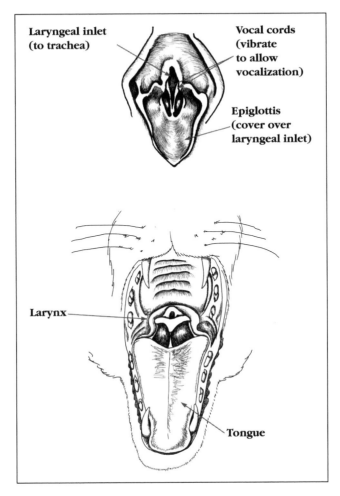

5-4 Larynx

may be excess salivation, and the body temperature may rise as the infection progresses.

What Are the Risks?
As with humans, most cases of laryngitis are not life threatening unless the infection spreads or breathing becomes severely impaired. Mild cases may simply run their course while more advanced cases will need treatment.

What Is the Treatment?
If the laryngitis persists or appears severe, a veterinary examination should be performed. This may require a tranquilizer. Most patients can be examined with a light called a laryngoscope. A culture can be

performed to help identify the organism responsible for the infection. Most viral causes simply run their course in 7 to 10 days. Bacterial or fungal causes can be treated with antibiotics or antifungals. Antihistamines such as Benadryl may be beneficial in some patients.

THE TRACHEA

The trachea is a long, hose-like tube that brings air through the neck and into the chest (see figure 5-5). It is also referred to as the **windpipe.** Once inside the chest, the trachea divides into two parts called the **bronchi.** One bronchi goes to the left lung; the other carries air to the right lung. The trachea contains cartilage rings that help keep it rigid as air moves in and out. Without these reinforcing cartilage rings, this tube structure would simply close if the cat took a deep breath.

TRACHEAL COLLAPSE

As mentioned earlier, a normal trachea is a rigid tube supported by rough rings made of cartilage. For unknown reasons, the cartilage rings sometimes begin to weaken and the trachea no longer has proper support. The trachea may lose its rigidity and collapse while the patient is breathing.

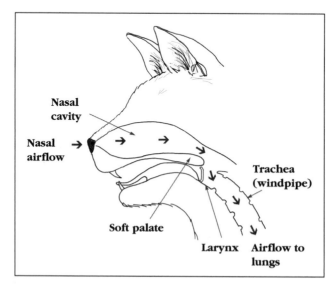

5-5 Upper respiratory system

What Are the Symptoms?

The symptoms of a collapsing trachea depend on the severity of the deterioration of the cartilage. Usually the patient will have difficulty breathing. The deeper the cat tries to inhale, the more the trachea collapses. This further restricts the air flow. This cat will usually appear to tire easily as it becomes short of breath. Patients with a collapsing trachea will generally cough as if trying to clear the airway. In very severe cases, the tongue and gums may appear blue as breathing becomes increasingly restricted.

What Is the Treatment?

Examination, whether by palpating with the fingers and/or the aid of radiographs (X-rays), will generally confirm the diagnosis. Depending on the severity, different medications can be used. Usually veterinarians prescribe drugs to help dilate the airways. Coughing may be decreased with cough suppressants such as Torbutrol. If the patient is obese, a strict diet is generally suggested. Activity should be restricted. This condition can be controlled but seldom cured, as nothing can restore the trachea's strength to normal levels. In very severe cases surgery can be performed to help open the airway and provide additional strength to its wall. Most cases, however, are managed medically, not surgically.

TRACHEOBRONCHITIS

Infections or irritations of the trachea and bronchi create a condition known as tracheobronchitis (see figure 5-6). As one might guess, coughing is the primary symptom associated with tracheobronchitis. Many disease-causing agents, whether bacterial, viral or fungal, can cause an infection within the trachea. The severity depends on the organism(s) involved.

What Are the Symptoms?

Most patients suffering from a tracheobronchitis exhibit coughing. They may even cough so severely that they regurgitate their food, leading the owner to believe the cat has an upset stomach, when in reality the stomach is normal. *Intestinal upsets do not begin with a cough.* Watch closely; if there is coughing until the cat vomits, the problem is in the trachea, not the stomach. The cough may also sound dry and raspy. Most patients act normal except they cough and occasionally gag. A fever may or may not be present.

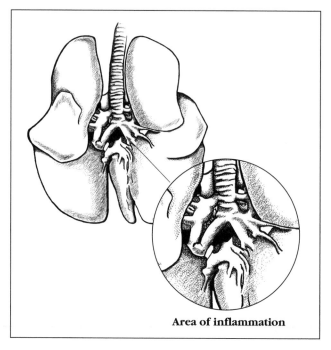

Area of inflammation

5-6   Tracheobronchitis

What Are the Risks?

If the infection is limited to the trachea, the risks are minimal. It must be noted, however, that many cases may take weeks to totally clear up. This is especially true of viral cases. Most cases of tracheobronchitis are extremely contagious. Although seldom life threatening, this disorder can certainly be a nuisance. In rare instances, the infection may spread to the lungs and create a more severe condition called pneumonia.

What Is the Treatment?

One must differentiate tracheobronchitis from the more serious pneumonitis. Occasionally, a patient may have both tracheobronchitis and pneumonitis. The tracheal manipulation test will help identify a patient with tracheobronchitis. If one takes a normal cat and gently grasps or puts pressure on the trachea in the neck, the cat will not cough. If however, the patient has an irritated trachea it will cough upon manipulation. Practitioners refer to this as a positive tracheal manipulation reflex. Listening to the lungs with a stethoscope will help identify a pneumonia. Patients with tracheobronchitis are generally placed on a cough suppressant such as Torbutrol. Medications to dilate the airways may also help alleviate the symptoms. Anti-inflammatories such as prednisone are commonly used to relieve the irritations. Antibiotics are useful if the causative agent is a bacteria.

LUNGS

The lungs are composed of millions of tiny spaces or air pockets called alveoli. It is here that fresh air from outside the body comes in close contact with a rich supply of small blood vessels known as capillaries. The blood exchanges carbon dioxide for oxygen and the red blood cells carry the oxygen to the tissues. This transfer of oxygen is absolutely essential to life. Any disease that upsets the delicate exchange of gases is potentially serious.

PNEUMONITIS

A lung infection or irritation is known as pneumonitis. If fluid builds up within the lung tissue, it is called pneumonia. *Pneumonia can occur after an infection; or may be secondary to another system failure, especially heart failure.* Disorders of the heart are described in Chapter 6. Infections of the lungs can be caused by bacteria, viruses or fungi. All can be serious. The most well-known cause of feline pneumonitis is the bacteria *Chlamydia psittaci.*

What Are the Symptoms?
The most frequent and noticeable symptom of a lung infection is difficult breathing, especially on inhalation. The breaths will be rapid and shallow. As the lung tissue becomes fluid-filled, the number of functional air spaces (alveoli) will be reduced. The patient has difficulties getting enough oxygen. The tongue, gums and lips may appear bluish or gray. This blue/gray appearance is termed cyanosis and is an indicator of a lack of oxygen within the blood. The body temperature is usually elevated, often to over 104 degrees Fahrenheit. If the lung congestion is caused by a failing heart, the temperature may remain within normal limits of 101 to 102 degrees Fahrenheit.

What Are the Risks?
Lung infections are always serious; however, with an early diagnosis and treatment most patients are treated successfully. In our opinion, the fungal diseases, such as blastomycosis, are some of the most serious. Early detection and an accurate diagnosis are very important. One must rely on the veterinarian to determine if the cause is heart-related or simply a primary infection of the lungs.

What Is the Treatment?
If one suspects a disorder of the lungs, a veterinarian should be contacted at once. A variety of diagnostic techniques such as chest radiographs (X-rays) or ultrasounds can be used. If fluid is suspected, the chest can

be biopsied so the material can be analyzed; this helps identify fungal disorders. If a bacteria is suspected, a culture and sensitivity can be performed to identify the bacterial type and help select the proper antibiotics. Diuretics, such as Lasix (Furosamide), are occasionally administered to help clear excess fluid from the lungs.

PNEUMOTHORAX

Pneumothorax is a term used to describe air within the chest cavity, but outside of the lungs. Remember that the areas in the chest surrounding the lungs are a vacuum allowing the easy expansion of the lungs during inhalation. Unwanted air can enter this vacuum in two ways. Any wound to the chest causing a puncture through the skin and chest wall will allow air into the vacuum. Secondly, trauma to the lungs can allow air to escape into the area around them. Broken ribs are sharp, and can puncture lung tissue, allowing air to leak from the lungs and into the surrounding chest cavity. Whatever the mechanism, once air enters the free area of the chest, the lungs are no longer supported by the vacuum and collapse to some degree.

What Are the Symptoms?

Generally, a pneumothorax will develop following chest trauma such as a puncture through the chest wall or a tearing of the lung tissue itself. Unless both sides of the chest cavity are damaged, usually only the right or the left lung is collapsed. The cat will have difficulty breathing, especially on inhalation. One will notice a rapid, shallow, difficult breathing rhythm. If the breathing is severely limited, the tongue, gums and lips may also appear blue. Severely wounded lungs may actually be exposed to the outside. Regardless of the degree of injury with a pneumothorax, the patient will be restless and try and lay in an upright position on the sternum. This position is known as *sternal recumbency.* This upright position helps the cat's lungs to be more easily inflated.

What Are the Risks?

The risks associated with a pneumothorax depend largely on the extent of the trauma. A simple puncture wound from a tooth may cause very little concern, while more severe lacerations can be immediately life threatening. *Do not assume, however, that a small puncture wound in the skin is not serious.* Often the underlying muscles are severely traumatized, and some ribs may also be broken. Chest wounds are easily contaminated. This can result in serious lung and chest infections. Since they are all potentially life threatening, have all chest wounds, no matter how slight, examined by a veterinarian at once.

What Is the Treatment?

The symptoms will not be alleviated until the chest wall is surgically repaired by closing the opening to the outside. Once the chest wall is repaired, the excess air is withdrawn from the chest cavity with a needle and syringe or a special valve. Antibiotics are generally administered to combat bacterial infections.

DIAPHRAGMATIC HERNIA

The large muscle that separates the chest and lungs from the liver and other abdominal organs is called the diaphragm. As the diaphragm contracts and relaxes, it enlarges and compresses the chest cavity; air is forced to move in and out of the lungs. The act of breathing depends largely on the function of the diaphragm muscle. Occasionally, the diaphragmatic muscle will become ruptured or torn. This typically follows a traumatic accident. Once an opening occurs within the muscle, abdominal contents such as the liver, stomach or intestines may herniate through the rupture, enter the chest and put pressure upon the lungs. The abilities of the diaphragm muscle are now compromised; it cannot properly expand and contract (see figure 5-7).

What Are the Symptoms?

Signs associated with diaphragmatic hernia may occur immediately after trauma or may not be noted for weeks. Difficulty breathing is the most common symptom. The degree depends on the extent of the damage and may vary from unnoticeable to extremely labored. In severe cases the tongue, lips and gums may appear bluish.

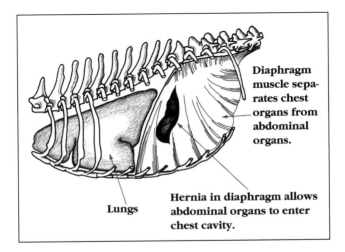

Diaphragm muscle separates chest organs from abdominal organs.

Lungs

Hernia in diaphragm allows abdominal organs to enter chest cavity.

5-7 Diaphragmatic hernia

Gastrointestinal upsets, such as vomiting or not eating, may also be noted when stomach or intestines herniate through the diaphragm. They become "strangulated" or pinched off by the muscle and other organs.

What Are the Risks?
The risks depend on the extent of the damage. Some patients with minor damage to the diaphragm actually go unnoticed and live normal lives. Patients with a severe injury to the diaphragm will quickly perish if left unattended.

What Is the Treatment?
Anytime this condition is suspected, a veterinarian should examine the patient at once. Radiographs (X-rays) will often lead to immediate diagnosis. Surgical correction is the only treatment of a diaphragmatic hernia, and it should be done as soon as the patient is stabilized.

LUNG CANCER

Tumors in the lungs are simply referred to as "lung cancer." Unlike humans, felines usually do not have tumors that originate within the lungs. In cats, the tumors are found elsewhere in the patient's body and they have merely spread (metastasized) to the lungs. As tumors grow, cancer cells tend to break away and float through the bloodstream. These cancer cells frequently lodge in the small vessels (capillaries) of the lungs and grow to form tumors. Eighty percent of all lung tumors of cats are termed *adenocarcinomas*. These are malignant (life-threatening) cancer growths that grow from abnormal glandular cells. Adenocarcinomas frequently originated from glandular tissues in the intestines, uterus or mammary glands. Skin and bone cancer may also spread to the lungs.

What Are the Symptoms?
The symptoms of lung cancer depend on the number and size of the tumors. The *one universal symptom is difficult breathing*. As the normal lung tissue is destroyed by the growing tumors, the patient tends to exhibit labored breathing that is rapid and shallow. Patients with lung cancer may also experience coughing, occasionally bringing up bloody mucous. In advanced cases, the patient will lose weight and eventually die. As mentioned earlier, other tissues in the cat are usually involved. Other symptoms depend on which other organs or areas of the body are also affected.

What Are the Risks?

Patients with lung cancer are seriously ill. Early detection and treatment may save or extend the lives of some patients, but most cases are incurable and die within six months.

What Is the Treatment?

As with humans, early detection and treatment is a must if the patient is to survive. Any cats with breathing difficulties should have a chest examination. This is generally done with the aid of a stethoscope and X-rays. Chest X-rays will frequently identify the number and sizes of the tumors. Ultrasound techniques are occasionally used. Once the tumors have been located, they can be surgically biopsied. Biopsies are obtained by opening up the chest and removing the tumors, or bypassing specialized biopsy needles through the chest wall and into the tumor to obtain some of the cancer cells. The biopsied material is then examined microscopically to determine the type of cancer. The treatment and outcome can then be predicted. Original tumors elsewhere in the body need to be dealt with for a complete cure.

The treatment varies greatly. Small tumors may simply be surgically removed. It is possible to surgically remove one or more lung lobes if needed. The cat can live with lung tissue on only one side, but activity would need to be restricted. In more severe instances chemotherapeutic drugs may be given. A few patients may be totally cured, but this is rare. In all likelihood, the cancer within the lungs originated from tumors elsewhere in the body. Both sites will need treatment in order to effect even a temporary cure.

A successful treatment may slow the tumor growth, thus extending the life span of the patient without ever providing a total cure. *The outcome is more promising if the cancer is detected in its early stages and treatment begins immediately.* It must be noted however, that ninety percent of all patients treated for lung cancer will die within a year. Without treatment, most die within six months. A thorough discussion of the condition between the veterinarian and the cat's owner is essential. Together they can decide the appropriate therapy and help predict the outcome.

FELINE ASTHMA (BRONCHIAL ASTHMA)

Bronchial asthma refers to a condition in which the airways become narrowed. The smooth muscle surrounding the airways, both the bronchi and bronchiolus, will spontaneously contract and therefore partially close the air passages. This is generally considered to be the result of an allergic response. Pollens, grasses and so on can all serve as allergens and trigger an acute bout of feline asthma. It is not currently known if allergies are the only factor that causes asthma, but they probably play a major role.

What Are the Symptoms?

A sudden attack of coughing is usually the initial sign of an asthma attack. As the airways constrict, the patient may have difficulty breathing. The mucous membranes of the mouth and tongue may appear cyanotic (blue) as adequate amounts of oxygen are not reaching the lungs and therefore the bloodstream. The symptoms are usually intermittent and the patient recovers and appears normal between attacks.

What Are the Risks?

The majority of asthmatic cats live normal life spans, but these cats are usually physically limited. Most have a decreased ability to exercise and appear lethargic or lazy. In severe instances, the asthma may progress to the point where adequate respiration becomes impossible and thereby the patient becomes severely limited.

What Is the Treatment?

Steroids, usually prednisone, are commonly used to suppress the allergic response. Bronchodilators such as Aminophylline are used to dilate or "open up" the air passages. In severe cases, oxygen therapy may be necessary. Steroids and bronchodilators are commonly administered throughout the life of the patient to help prevent the asthma attacks.

CHAPTER 6

The Heart, Vessels and Blood (The Circulatory System)

The feline circulatory system is much like the human's. The **heart** has *four chambers;* the two upper chambers are the *left and right atria,* while the stronger, lower chambers are the *right and left ventricles* (see figure 6-1). Blood travels from the tissues and enters the right **atrium.** From there it moves into the right **ventricle.** The right ventricle pumps blood from the body into the lungs, where oxygen is exchanged for carbon dioxide produced by cellular metabolism. Blood, now rich in oxygen, leaves the lungs via the pulmonary vein and enters the left atrium. The left atrium pumps blood to the left ventricle, the most heavily muscled and strongest of the chambers. The left ventricle pumps blood to the great aorta, which supplies the body with blood and oxygen. The chambers are separated by muscle and a series of valves (see figure 6-2). The **tricuspid valve** separates the right atrium and right ventricle, while the **mitral valve** separates the left atrium from the left ventricle. In order for the heart to pump efficiently, each chamber and valve must function in a coordinated effort.

Blood is comprised of several different types of cells and proteins. **Red blood cells** give blood its color and are responsible for the transportation of both oxygen and carbon dioxide to and from the body's tissues. **White blood cells** fight infection. A third cell type, the **platelets,** circulate in the blood and are responsible for clotting. Platelets, white blood cells and red blood cells are formed in the bone marrow. In addition to cells, the blood is made up of a protein-rich liquid called plasma.

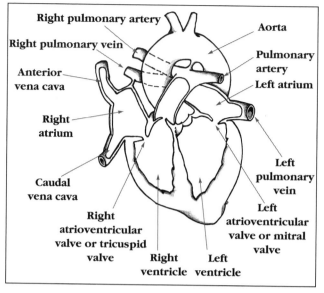

6-1 Feline heart

CARDIOMYOPATHY

Cardiomyopathy is a term used to describe a diseased heart muscle. *In cats, the majority of heart diseases affect the muscles of the heart rather than the valves or vessels.* The two most commonly encountered cardiomyopathies are *congestive,* or dilated, and *hypertrophic.*

In congestive cardiomyopathy, also known as dilated cardiomyopathy, the heart muscles become thin and weakened. The muscle of the left ventricle is the most affected and will have a very poor contractability. The heart will appear rounded and soft, much like a balloon. Because the muscle is thin and weak, blood is not efficiently pumped from the left ventricle into the aorta and out to the body.

Hypertrophic cardiomyopathy is a condition in which the heart muscles become thickened; it's the opposite of congestive cardiomyopathy. The walls of the left ventricle become so thick that the left heart chamber is "crowded out" and becomes smaller than normal.

Although hypertrophic and congestive cardiomyopathy appear to be nearly opposite in cause, the end results are similar. In both instances the left ventricle cannot pump enough blood to the body. Patients of all ages may be involved, but those most at risk are the middle-aged and elderly.

What Are the Symptoms?

Cardiomyopathy, regardless of cause or type, is a disease of the heart muscles. Because of varying degrees in severity and exact areas of the

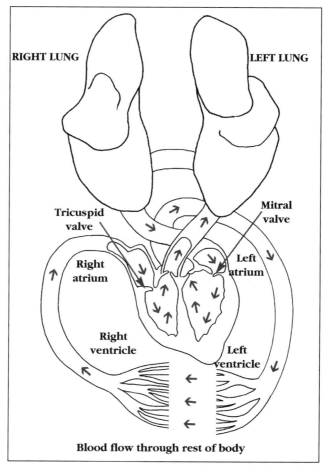

6-2   Heart and blood flow

heart involved, there can be many symptoms. Most commonly (regardless of cause), the patient will have decreased stamina, and upon exercise, the patient may experience a lack of adequate oxygen because of the heart's inability to pump efficiently. Fainting episodes may occur as a result of inadequate oxygen. Fluid may accumulate in the lungs, causing coughing and/or labored breathing. Additionally, fluid may build up in the abdomen, causing the cat to become bloated. Murmurs, along with an abnormal heart rate and rhythm, may also be present. Occasionally, with no warning signs, a patient suddenly collapses and dies of a heart attack due to cardiomyopathy.

What Are the Risks?

Whenever the heart muscles are diseased, the condition is serious. The levels of severity of cardiomyopathy pose different risks. In some patients the signs are slow in development and progression, while sudden death may occur in other patients.

What Is the Treatment?

Many cardiac patients can be helped with medications, although with cardiomyopathy a complete cure usually is not possible. Various drugs are available to help strengthen the contractions of the heart muscles in the patient with congestive cardiomyopathy. Diuretics or water pills are used to help remove excess fluid from the lungs and abdomen.

The exact treatment depends on a careful evaluation of the patient. Factors such as which type of cardiomyopathy exists, severity of the condition, the cat's age and so on are taken into consideration when developing a treatment strategy. Diagnostics such as EKGs, X-rays (radiographs), echocardiograms and venous dye studies (angiograms) may all help produce an accurate diagnosis and treatment plan.

VEGETATIVE ENDOCARDITIS

Bacteria occasionally enter the bloodstream. From there they can be carried to the heart and cause an infection. An endocarditis is an infection of the heart. The term "vegetative" arises from the fact that when bacteria colonize an area of the heart such as the valves, the diseased areas grow and take on a vegetable-like appearance. Bacterially infected heart tissue actually resembles the head of a cauliflower. The heart valves are particularly susceptible to damage if bacteria infect the heart.

What Are the Symptoms?

The symptoms of a vegetative endocarditis are not always clearly defined. Intermittent fevers may be the only sign. In advanced cases, weight loss, heart murmurs and anemia may be detected.

What Are the Risks?

An infection of the heart is serious and life threatening. Early detection and treatment is necessary to reduce the risk of damage to the heart.

What Is the Treatment?

Since most cases are caused by a bacteria, antibiotics are the treatment of choice. A blood culture may be necessary to help identify the bacteria involved. More than one month of continuous antibiotic therapy may be needed. Treatment must be vigorous to be successful.

ARTERIAL THROMBOEMBOLISM (SADDLE THROMBI)

Thromboembolism, or blood clot formation, is much more common in the feline than in the canine. Blood clots originating in the heart will be released into the aorta where they will travel through the aorta

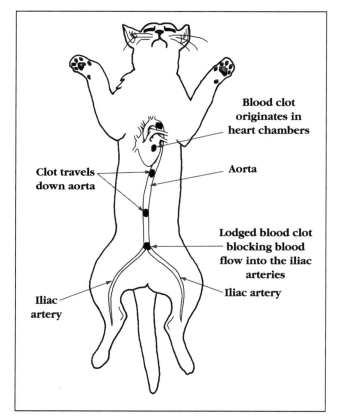

**Blood clot
originates in
heart chambers**

**Clot travels
down aorta**

Aorta

**Lodged blood clot
blocking blood
flow into the iliac
arteries**

Iliac artery

**Iliac
artery**

6-3   Saddle thrombi

branches into the iliac arteries. The iliac arteries, located in the abdomen, are the most common area for the clot(s) to lodge (see figure 6-3). The iliac arteries supply oxygenated blood to the rear limbs; when a blood clot is obstructing blood flow to the legs, the rear limb muscles are unable to function. It is not known why the clots occur; however, they are most common in cats with a cardiomyopathy.

What Are the Symptoms?

The symptoms associated with a saddle thrombi are not easily confused with other disorders; they are quite specific. Within minutes of the blood clot obstruction, the iliac arteries of the cat become severely blocked, causing paralysis in the rear limbs. There will be no detectable pulse in the hind legs. Initially, the cat is in extreme discomfort. This pain is most likely due to the lack of oxygen to the hind leg muscles. The rear legs will feel cold to the touch, and the toenail beds will be blue rather than pink. There are cases in which one hind limb is more affected than the other; and some patients experience partial obstruction. In both these scenarios the symptoms may be less severe.

What Are the Risks?

A complete, irreversible paralysis may be the result. A partial obstruction from a small clot will have a better outcome than a complete blockage. The majority of the cats treated by the authors continued to develop additional clots. To reduce the risk of a permanent paralysis, it is imperative that treatment be administered at once. *This is an emergency situation.*

What Is the Treatment?

Drugs to dissolve the clot and restore blood flow to the limbs are used with occasionally excellent results. Such drugs include Heparin, aspirin, and Coumarin. Surgery to remove the clot has also been successful in some patients, but pharmaceutical treatment is usually preferred.

HEART AND VESSEL BIRTH DEFECTS

The fetus gets its blood supply from the mother through the umbilical cord. The lungs serve no function until birth, at which time the kitten is exposed to breathable air. Blood in the fetus, therefore, bypasses the lungs and flows directly from the right heart chambers to the left chambers via a vessel called the ductus arteriosus. At birth, the ductus arteriosus closes off permanently, forcing blood to flow through the lungs for the oxygen/carbon dioxide exchange. Similarly within the fetus, vessels bypass the liver until birth. The fetus depends on the mother's liver to provide needed functions. At birth, the vessels close and the infant's blood is then routed through the kitten's liver.

ATRIOVENTRICULAR VALVE COMPLEX MALFORMATION

This is the most common heart defect in the cat. The mitral valve separates the left atrium from the left ventricle. The tricuspid valve separates the right atrium from the right ventricle (see figure 6-4). If the valve(s) and its muscles do not develop properly (such as forming a valve(s) that doesn't completely open or close), the result will be an abnormal flow of blood between the heart chambers.

What Are the Symptoms?

Most severely affected cats are less than one year of age when symptoms develop. Common signs include failure to grow (usually referred to as stunted growth), lethargy, difficulty breathing and coughing due to a fluid buildup in the lungs. A murmur is usually detectable with the aid of a stethoscope. In some instances the heart murmur is the only detectable symptom.

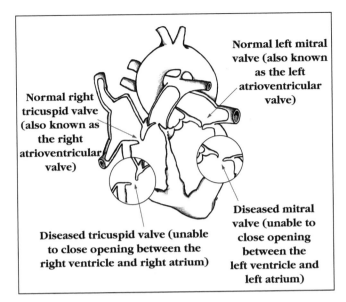

Normal left mitral valve (also known as the left atrioventricular valve)

Normal right tricuspid valve (also known as the right atrioventricular valve)

Diseased tricuspid valve (unable to close opening between the right ventricle and right atrium)

Diseased mitral valve (unable to close opening between the left ventricle and left atrium)

6-4   Normal and diseased tricuspid and mitral valves

What Are the Risks?

This heart defect is serious and the patient may die of cardiac failure. If the defects are severe, the heart may wear out at a very young age. It is possible, however, for some cats with mildly affected valves to live relatively normal lives. This is true even when a detectable heart murmur is present.

What Is the Treatment?

EKGs (electrocardiograms), echocardiograms, radiographs and so on are frequently used to characterize the valve defects and help determine the benefits of treatment. If treatment is elected, it involves surgery to replace the abnormal valves.

PATENT DUCTUS ARTERIOSUS (PDA)

As stated earlier, the ductus arteriosus allows blood to bypass the lungs in the fetus (see figure 6-5). The lungs are not yet needed for breathing, so blood simply flows through the ductus arteriosus, bypassing the lungs. At birth, due to pressure changes within the bloodstream, the ductus closes permanently, forcing blood to now enter the lungs where carbon dioxide can be exchanged for oxygen. In the cases of a patent ductus arteriosus (PDA), the vessel fails to completely close and some blood continues to bypass the lungs. When this happens, even though the kitten is breathing, the proper amount of blood is not flowing to the lungs and the kitten is not receiving enough oxygen to meet the tissue demands.

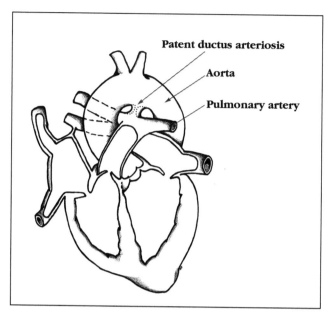

6-5 Patent ductus arteriosis (PDA)

What Are the Symptoms?

Initially, the kitten may show no symptoms. As it grows, however, the circulatory system cannot keep up with the tissues' demand for oxygen. As the kitten grows and the oxygen demands are not met, the kitten may compensate for the oxygen deficit by becoming less active. A kitten at rest will require less oxygen than one at play. Inactivity is one of the initial signs of PDA. In periods of excitement these kittens may collapse as they become short of breath. The gums will appear bluish (cyanotic), reflecting the oxygen shortage. As the blood flows through the abnormal ductus arteriosus, a murmur caused by turbulent blood flow can sometimes be heard without the aid of a stethoscope. This abnormal blood flow can occasionally be felt if one palpates the chest. Depending on the severity, the signs may first be noted anywhere in the first year of life. Many affected kittens will not grow at a normal rate and will be smaller than their littermates.

What Are the Risks?

Without treatment, almost all patients with a PDA will have a shortened life span. Depending on severity, some will live only a few weeks, while others may survive longer.

What Is the Treatment?

Treatment of a PDA requires surgery. The surgical procedure involves tying off the ductus arteriosus with suture material, thus routing all of the blood flow through the lungs. Surgery is quite successful and is best if done early, before growth is affected.

VENTRICULAR SEPTAL DEFECT (VSD)

In the developing embryo, the heart initially has four chambers that are not separated from one another. As the fetal heart develops, walls called septums form to divide the heart into four separate chambers. Occasionally the walls separating the heart chambers will not develop completely, and the chambers will not be properly divided from each other. This congenital birth defect is commonly referred to as a "hole in the heart." In reality there is no hole in the heart, but rather a hole *between* the heart chambers (see figure 6-6). This septal defect typically occurs between the right and left ventricles, hence the name **v**entricular **s**eptal **d**efect (VSD).

What Are the Symptoms?

Because the left ventricle is stronger than the right ventricle, blood is forced backward against the normal flow patterns. Whenever this occurs, an additional work load is placed on these structures, possibly leading to heart failure. Additionally with VSD, inadequate quantities of oxygenated blood are supplied to the body tissues.

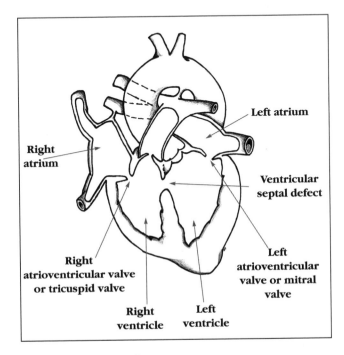

6-6   Ventricular septal defect (VSD)

Patients may not exhibit any outward signs of VSD. Occasionally, upon a routine examination, veterinarians listening with a stethoscope will hear the heart murmur associated with VSD. In severe septal defects, a decrease in stamina and retarded growth rates occur.

What Are the Risks?

Many patients with minor septal defects live normal lives even though a heart murmur is detectable. Occasionally, the septal defect closes spontaneously as late as two years of age. Patients with large septal defects typically have a shortened life span, generally succumbing to heart failure.

What Is the Treatment?

In minor septal defects, treatment is generally not recommended. In severe instances, heart surgery can be performed to correct the defect.

AORTIC STENOSIS

The great vessel called the aorta carries blood from the left side of the heart to all organs and tissues of the body. Occasionally, a narrowing of the aorta or its valves will be present. This is a developmental congenital defect that retards normal blood flow out the aorta. To compensate for this, the left side of the heart enlarges as it is pumping against increased resistance. The left side of the heart becomes overworked.

What Are the Symptoms?

Most affected patients have a low level of activity. They tire easily upon exercise, and occasionally a patient may pass out due to lack of oxygen in the tissues. A cat with aortic stenosis generally appears weak.

What Are the Risks?

Aortic stenosis is a serious condition and sudden death can occur. Patients with an overworked heart often die from heart failure before reaching two years of age.

What Is the Treatment?

Surgery does not usually produce good results; and medications also have met with little success. Most patients go untreated.

PORTAL CAVAL SHUNT

The liver in the developing fetus is bypassed by vessels that shunt blood around it. As long as the fetus exchanges blood with the mother, the fetal liver functions are minimal and an extensive blood flow is not needed. A portal caval shunt describes a situation in which some or all of the blood vessels bypassing the liver do not degenerate prior to birth. Because some of the blood vessels maintain their embryonic patterns, the blood continues to flow around the liver tissue and not through it.

The liver is responsible for several important functions (see Chapter 3). It removes wastes and toxins from the bloodstream, stores materials such as glucose and fats, and it forms and stores vitamins. It also produces various enzymes and proteins that aid in digestion. In a portal caval shunt, none of these tasks are performed at their appropriate level.

What Are the Symptoms?

Most clinical signs of portal caval shunt are related to the buildup of toxins within the bloodstream. These toxins are normal by-products of cellular metabolism, but in high concentrations they act like poisons in the body. Symptoms may develop anytime during the first six months of life. Since these poisons are building within the bloodstream, they affect other organs such as the brain. The term "hepatic encephalopathy" is used to describe a patient having neurological signs caused by toxic effects of metabolic wastes on the brain. The buildup of metabolic toxins can cause poor appetite, dizziness, seizures, blindness, staggering, lethargy, depression and stupor.

What Are the Risks?

The risks are great and early death is common. As the animal grows, the symptoms worsen. The increase in body size means more cells are producing metabolic by-products and these same cells are in greater need of products formed or stored by a normal liver.

What Is the Treatment?

The neurologic symptoms are treated with anticonvulsant drugs to prevent seizures. Medications can help to control the condition, but often they are not a cure. Generally, restricted protein diets minimize the buildup of nitrogen waste in the bloodstream. Surgery, the only true cure, is required to close off the vessels bypassing the liver.

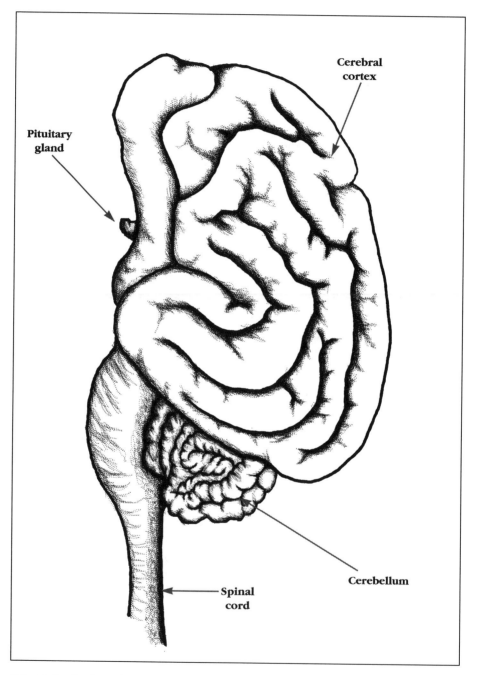

7-1 Feline brain and pituitary gland

C H A P T E R   7

Hormone Disorders

The **endocrine glands** produce chemicals called hormones. When hormones other than prostaglandins enter the bloodstream, they affect cells elsewhere in the body. Not all cells within the body are affected by hormones, and some cells of a particular organ may respond only to a *specific* hormone.

Some hormones control the release of other hormones. For example, the **pituitary gland** located at the base of the brain (see figure 7-1) produces many hormones. These hormones act on other glands, such as the **adrenals,** by prompting them to release their own hormones. *The pituitary gland* is called *"the master gland,"* as it provides more *kinds* of hormones than any other gland. *Pituitary hormones* control the hormone release of other endocrine glands, including the **thyroid, parathyroid, adrenal, ovaries, testicles** and **pancreas.**

The pituitary gland produces a *growth hormone*, which controls growth; the *prolactin hormone,* which stimulates the mammary glands to produce milk; the *thyroid-stimulating hormone (TSH)*, which stimulates the thyroid gland; and the *luteinizing hormone (LH)* and *follicle-stimulating hormone (FSH)*, which control heat cycles and ovulation. The pituitary gland also produces *adrenocorticotropic hormone (ACTH)*, which in turn causes the adrenal gland to produce cortisol and other hormones, and the *melanocyte-stimulating hormone (MSH)*, which affects pigment.

The **thyroid gland,** once stimulated, produces its own hormone, *thyroxine.* The **ovaries,** when stimulated by FSH and LH from the pituitary, principally produce *progesterone* and *estrogens.* The **testes** provide *testosterone.* The **pancreas** produces the most well-known hormone of all: *insulin,* which regulates blood sugar. Once stimulated by the pituitary hormone ACTH, the **adrenal glands** produce naturally occurring steroids called *corticosteroids, mineralocorticoids* and *adrenal sex*

97

steroids. Contrary to popular belief, steroids are found naturally in the body. Pharmaceutically manufactured steroids, such as cortisones, are available for use in pets. Pet owners are often concerned about the side effects of steroids, and certainly there are some; however, steroids are absolutely essential for life.

As one can see, hormones play a very complex role in regulating the body's functions. This chapter will discuss only those hormone conditions commonly encountered in veterinary medicine.

DISORDERS OF THE PANCREAS

The pancreas is a gray, ribbon-like gland located adjacent to the stomach and small intestine (see figure 7-2). It has two major functions: it produces enzymes to aid in digestion, and it produces hormones to control blood sugar (glucose) levels.

In this chapter, we are concerned with its production of hormones, insulin and glucagon. The production of digestive enzymes is discussed in Chapter 3, "The Digestive Organs—Liver, Pancreas and Gallbladder."

When starches and carbohydrates are eaten, they are broken down into the sugar glucose. This is absorbed through the wall of the digestive tract where it passes into the bloodstream. Insulin allows glucose to leave the bloodstream and enter the body's tissue. It is used as energy for the cells. When glucose levels are high, glucagon causes it to be stored in the liver and muscles as glycogen.

DIABETES MELLITUS ("SUGAR" DIABETES)

Diabetes mellitus, commonly referred to simply as diabetes, is a condition in which the pancreas does not produce sufficient quantities of the hormone insulin. Insulin is necessary to move glucose into the cells from the bloodstream. Brain cells, as well as intestinal and red blood cells, do not need high levels of insulin for glucose transport across their walls. However, the body tissues need glucose for energy. With diabetes, the glucose simply builds up in the bloodstream, causing an elevated blood sugar level.

What Are the Symptoms?

Elevated blood sugar (glucose) can affect many body systems. Excess blood sugar will be lost through the kidneys, causing increased urination and thirst. Elevated blood sugar also alters the lens of the eye, leading to diabetic cataracts. Weight loss is a common symptom as the body burns muscle for energy to help compensate for the body's

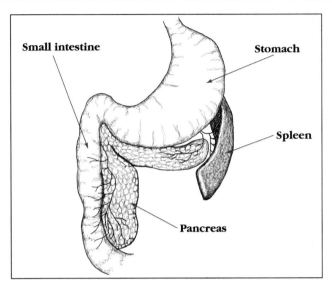

7-2 Pancreas

inability to use glucose. A loss of muscle mass combined with inadequate energy levels within the cells leads to generalized weakness. The most common signs of diabetes are weakness, weight loss and increased thirst and urination.

What Are the Risks?
The elevated blood sugar is toxic to many body systems and organs, including the blood vessels, nervous system (brain), liver, etc. A patient with uncontrolled diabetes will not live a normal life span. At the first indication of diabetes, a blood test should be performed by a veterinarian to determine the blood sugar level. The earlier treatment is initiated, the better.

What Is the Treatment?
Unlike with humans, simply controlling the diet is seldom beneficial in the feline. Oral insulin tablets are not commonly effective in pets. The treatment for a diabetic feline usually involves daily insulin injections. Patients must be carefully monitored with blood and urine sugar tests to help determine the proper amount of insulin. Daily feeding must be on a regular schedule to provide a consistent supply of sugar so that insulin remains at the required level.

  With proper care most patients with diabetes can live relatively normal lives. Maintaining the diabetic pet requires dedication on the part of the owner. Many pet owners have found this to be a rewarding experience.

DISORDERS OF THE ADRENALS

The body has two adrenal glands, one located next to each kidney (see figure 7-3). In the feline, adrenal glands are slightly smaller than a BB. The **medulla,** the inner core of the glands, secretes the hormones *adrenaline* (epinephrine) and *noradrenaline* (norepinephrine). These two hormones control blood pressure and heart rate. The outer shell of the adrenal glands is called the **cortex.** This secretes the *corticosteroid* and *sex steroid hormones.* There are two types of corticosteroids: the mineralocorticoids and the glucocorticoids. *Aldosterone* is a mineralocorticoid that regulates the amount of sodium lost in the urine. *Hydrocortisone* (cortisol), a glucocorticoid hormone, helps control the metabolism of carbohydrates. The sex steroids produced by the adrenal cortex are also referred to as the sex hormones. These are *androgens* and *estrogens.*

CUSHING'S DISEASE

Cushing's disease (or syndrome) results when the adrenal glands overproduce steroid hormones. This may be caused by disease in either the adrenal glands, the pituitary gland (which stimulates the adrenal glands) or the hypothalamus (a section of the brain that stimulates the pituitary gland). Additionally, an artificial Cushing's syndrome can be seen if a patient is being given excessive levels of steroid medication. Tumors of the hypothalamus, pituitary or adrenal gland can cause overproduction of steroid hormones, resulting in Cushing's disease.

What Are the Symptoms?
The body of a cat with Cushing's disease typically will appear puffy from weight gain. Fatty deposits accumulate under the skin and within the body cavities due to uncontrolled metabolism of carbohydrates. Additionally, the skin over the abdomen and flank area will become thin and may contain small, white mineral (calcium) deposits. Muscle mass and strength are lost. The patient will develop a "pot-bellied" appearance as the abdominal muscles become weak. The legs will appear spindly, and the animal may have problems getting up or jumping on furniture. Thirst and appetite will usually be excessive.

What Are the Risks?
Cushing's disease is often caused by cancer of the hypothalamus, pituitary or adrenal glands. The first two are adjacent to the brain. Any tumors in this area have potentially serious consequences. *Cushing's disease is serious and, without treatment, usually fatal.*

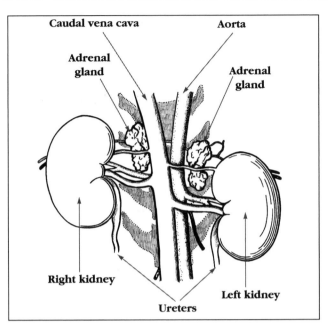

7-3   Feline adrenal glands

What Is the Treatment?

The cause must be determined. If the patient is receiving excessive steroid medication for another condition, then merely altering the dosage may correct the problem. If your cat is on steroids for a medical condition, always consult your veterinarian before increasing or decreasing the dose.

Surgery may be needed if diagnostic tests reveal a tumor. Drugs are also available that can destroy portions of the adrenal gland, thus reducing the abnormally high hormonal output.

ADDISON'S DISEASE

Addison's disease describes a patient with underactive adrenal glands. Occasionally due to age or damage from infections or drug therapy, the adrenal cortex will not produce enough steroid hormones.

What Are the Symptoms?

Weight loss, anemia, diarrhea, loss of appetite and vomiting can all be signs of Addison's disease.

What Are the Risks?

Fluid loss along with mineral imbalances create a serious situation. Left untreated, the cat with Addison's will experience dehydration and death.

What Is the Treatment?

Diagnostic blood tests to check sodium and potassium levels will help confirm a diagnosis of Addison's. Medications such as Florinef can be administered to replace the inadequate hormones. Most patients respond very well to therapy.

DISORDERS OF THE THYROID

The thyroid gland consists of two lobes located near the larynx (Adam's apple) in the cat's neck (see figure 7-4). The thyroid gland combines the amino acid tyrosine and iodine to manufacture the thyroid hormone. The pituitary gland exerts control over the thyroid gland. TSH from the pituitary stimulates the thyroid gland to produce its hormone, thyroxine. Thyroxine is the hormone that controls metabolic and activity levels. The thyroid gland also secretes another hormone, calcitonin, which is necessary for proper calcium metabolism. An underactive thyroid, or *hypo*thyroidism, is very rare in the cat. An overactive thyroid, or *hyper*thyroidism, is more common. The opposite is true of the canine.

HYPERTHYROIDISM

In contrast to the canine, hyperthyroidism, or an *overactive* thyroid gland, is fairly common in the feline. The most common cause of an overactive thyroid is a tumor called an adenoma. The adenoma arises as a growth from the thyroid gland. The tumor, being comprised of thyroid gland cells, will secrete excessive quantities of the thyroid hormone, thyroxine.

What Are the Symptoms?

Usually, a cat with hyperthyroidism will have a normal to voracious appetite. Due to the excess levels of thyroxine, the patient often is hyperactive and *loses* weight despite a ravenous appetite. Following the increased appetite is the production of more feces, resulting in increased defecation. The heart rate will be increased and may rise to as much as double the normal rate.

What Are the Risks?

A mild case of hyperthyroidism will initially present little if any problem. As the tumor grows, the excess levels of thyroxine will become very high. Left untreated, the patient may die due to excessive weight loss and/or the heart simply wearing out.

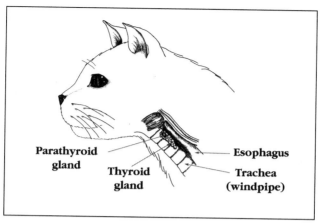

7-4   Thyroid and parathyroid glands

What Is the Treatment?

Surgery may be performed to remove the adenoma and excess glandular tissue. This will lower the thyroxine production. Drugs are available that will selectively target and destroy thyroid glandular tissue. Radiation therapy to destroy thyroid tissue has also been used.

Of the three above treatments, surgery is the most popular. Whatever the treatment used, it is not possible to remove or destroy the *exact* amount of glandular cells. Following treatment, the patient is usually left with an *underactive* thyroid or *hypo*thyroidism. A daily supplementation of thyroid hormone in pill form can now be added to bring the hormone level back into the normal range.

PRIMARY HYPERPARATHYROIDISM

This describes an overactive parathyroid gland that produces too much parathyroid hormone, thus increasing the blood calcium levels. Calcium is selectively removed from the bones, causing them to soften. Hyperparathyroidism is not common in the cat, but is the most common disorder affecting the feline parathyroid gland.

What Are the Symptoms?

In most cases no visible symptoms are present; however, routine blood tests may detect a high level of blood calcium.

What Are the Risks?

In the long term, bones will become soft and may fracture at the slightest injury. Kidney and/or bladder stones may form as a result of the altered calcium levels.

What Is the Treatment?

This condition is usually caused by tumors in the parathyroid glands. Surgery to remove the growths will lower the hormone production.

OTHER HORMONAL DISORDERS

DIABETES INSIPIDUS

Diabetes insipidus is the result of an underproduction of the anti-diuretic hormone (ADH) by the hypothalamus. The hypothalamus is an area of the brain immediately adjacent to the pituitary gland. Once secreted into the blood, ADH or the anti-diuretic hormone travels to the kidney where it causes the kidney to conserve or retain water for the body.

What Are the Symptoms?

The patient with diabetes insipidus lacks proper levels of the hormone ADH, which allows the kidneys to conserve water. A patient with inadequate anti-diuretic hormone will lose water in the urine and attempt to compensate by drinking more. Excessive thirst and urination are the principal symptoms.

What Are the Risks?

Mild cases only cause the cat to drink and urinate excessive amounts of water. More severe cases will cause the patient to dehydrate to the point of death.

What Is the Treatment?

There is no treatment for diabetes insipidus. Fortunately, it is not common. It is included in this text to help differentiate the two forms of diabetes—diabetes insipidus and diabetes mellitus. *Although the names are similar, the disorders are very different.*

FELINE ENDOCRINE ALOPECIA

Feline endocrine alopecia is a loss of hair due to a hormone imbalance. The exact hormones involved are not always known; however, the sex steroids such as testosterone, estrogens and progesterones are known to play a role. An imbalance of these hormones is usually the cause.

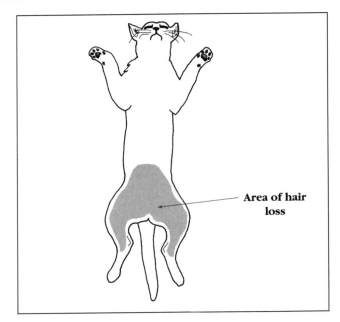

Area of hair loss

7-5 Feline endocrine alopecia

What Are the Symptoms?

A loss of hair on the inner thighs, belly and inguinal area is the most common sign (see figure 7-5). Male cats, especially those neutered at an immature age, seem to have the highest incidence. It does, however, occur in females and is more common in those that have been spayed.

What Are the Risks?

Although the loss of hair is evident, the disease is not serious. It is important to recognize this as a hair loss disorder so that it can be distinguished from other causes such as allergies, flea infestations and psychogenic alopecia. (See Chapter 11, "The Skin, Hair and Nails.")

What Is the Treatment?

Most patients respond favorably to an oral dose of megestrol acetate. This is a hormone-replacement medication commonly available through veterinarians under the names of Ovaban or Megace. Long-term therapy of Ovaban given once or twice weekly may be required.

The hair coat usually returns to normal after several months of therapy. Due to the potential side effects of megestrol acetate, a careful evaluation of the patient should be made to determine if treatment is necessary.

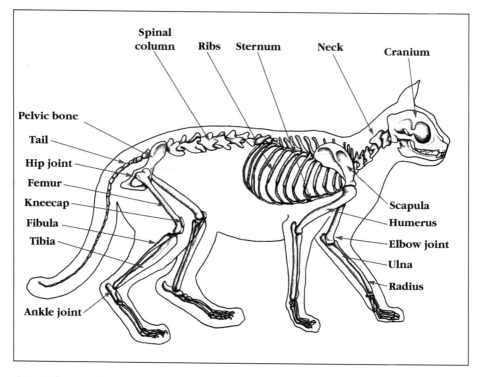

Spinal
column   Ribs   Sternum   Neck   Cranium

Pelvic bone

Tail

Hip joint

Femur

Kneecap

Fibula

Tibia

Scapula

Humerus

Elbow joint

Ulna

Radius

Ankle joint

8-1   Feline anatomy

CHAPTER 8

Bones, Joints, Muscles, Ligaments and Tendons (The Musculoskeletal System)

The skeletal system and its interconnecting tissues—the **muscles, ligaments** and **tendons**—form the bulk of the cat's body mass. The bones are connected by complex areas of articulation. Each of these areas form a joint.

Allowing for variations, there are more than 210 bones in the feline skeleton (see figure 8-1). Variations exist primarily because of differing tail lengths (see figure 8-2). Bones are complex, rigid, living organs that have their own supply of blood vessels and nerves.

Bones are composed of minerals and are high in calcium and phosphorus. Bones provide both the body framework and the protection for many delicate internal organs and structures. For example, the bones of the skull protect the brain and eyes, while the breast plate (sternum) helps protect the heart and lungs. Other bones, such as those of the limbs, function to provide support and locomotion. Bones of the internal ear structure function for neither protection nor support, but rather they transmit sound, which allows the cat to hear.

Muscles function primarily to move all or part of the cat's body. *Smooth muscles* are found within the internal organs, such as the intestines, stomach and bladder. These are not subject to voluntary or conscious control by the individual. They work automatically to satisfy the body's needs. *Striated muscles* are predominately attached to the skeleton. All of their movements are under the conscious control of the individual. They are involved with such activities as walking, eating, moving the tail, moving the eyes and so on. The skeletal or striated muscles will be discussed in the remainder of this chapter.

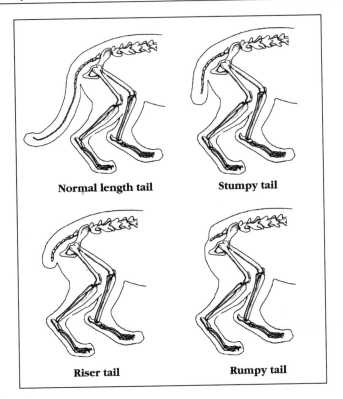

Normal length tail

Stumpy tail

Riser tail

Rumpy tail

8-2 Tail lengths

One half of the cat's total weight is skeletal muscle. Skeletal muscles are connected to the bones by tough, fibrous bands called **tendons.** Tendons begin on a muscle and end on a bone. A good example is the Achilles tendon, which connects the muscle of the calf (lower rear limb) to the bones forming the ankle (see figure 8-3). Another important function of tendons in the cat is extending and retracting the claws (see figure 8-4).

Ligaments connect bone to bone and are generally found bridging the joints. Joints are places where two bones meet or articulate; their ends are covered by a layer of smooth cartilage. Joints consist of bones, muscles, ligaments, cartilage and a lubricating joint fluid all enclosed by a tough joint capsule (see figure 8-5). A joint by itself is not considered an organ.

DISORDERS OF THE BONES AND JOINTS

Bones and joints can be damaged or become diseased. Even normal aging can have a profound effect on the joints. Arthritis is an example of a disease that can be a normal component of aging.

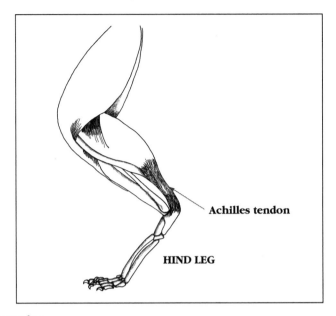

8-3   Achilles tendon

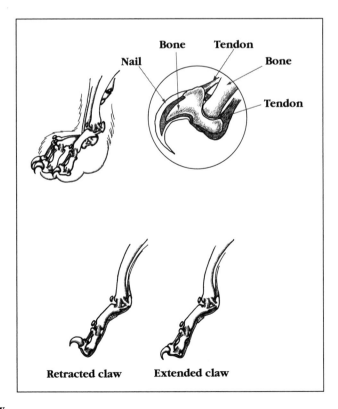

8-4   Cat paw

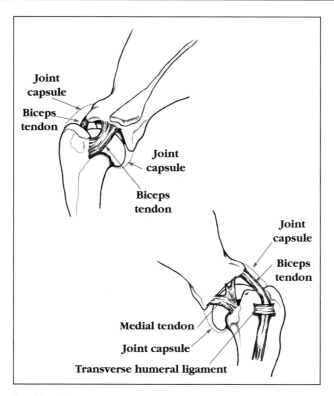

8-5   Feline shoulder joint

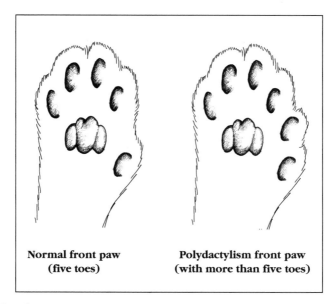

8-6   Polydactylism

POLYDACTYLISM

Polydactyly refers to a cat with an above average number of toes. Normal cats have five toes on each front foot and four on each rear foot. The front feet are much more likely to have extra toes than the rear (see figure 8-6). Polydactyly is an inherited condition.

What Are the Symptoms?
By definition, a cat with more than five toes on a front foot or four on each rear foot is a polydactyl cat.

What Are the Risks?
Although the extra toes are referred to as abnormal, polydactyl cats are normal. They simply carry the genes for polydactylism. The main concern is the size of the feet. The toenails do not always wear evenly, and therefore excess nail growth is not uncommon.

Occasionally, the nails will grow to the extent that they curl around and grow into the pads. We refer to this as ingrown nails. Infections can develop as a result of ingrown nails.

What Is the Treatment?
The extra toes are normal and should not be removed. To prevent ingrown toenails, it is often necessary to clip or trim the nails. Cat nails grow rapidly and may need trimming every month to prevent excessive growth.

OPEN FONTANELS

Please see Hydrocephaly in Chapter 9, "The Nervous System."

LUXATED PATELLAS

The bone we know as the kneecap is also referred to as the patella. A groove in the lower (distal) femur allows the patella to glide up and down when the knee joint is bent back and forth. In so doing, it guides the action of the quadricep muscle to the lower leg. The patella or knee cap also provides bony protection for the knee joint.

Occasionally, because of malformation or trauma the ridges forming the patellar groove are not prominent, and a groove that is too shallow is created. In a patient with shallow grooves, the patella will dislocate (luxate) sideways, typically to the middle (medial) side. This causes the leg to "lock up" with the foot held up off the ground. One or both knees may be involved. All breeds are susceptible to patella luxation;

however, the Devon Rex has a higher incidence, suggesting that genetics plays a role.

What Are the Symptoms?

Most patients are middle-aged. They present a history of intermittent lameness on the affected rear leg(s). Patients commonly stop and cry out in pain as they are running. Their legs will be extended rearward, and they are unable to flex them back into the normal position. The patella has actually flipped sideways outside the groove preventing the leg from bending correctly. Most commonly, only one leg is affected.

What Are the Risks?

Left untreated, the patellar ridges will wear incorrectly, causing the groove to become even more shallow. The patient will become progressively more lame. Arthritis will prematurely affect the joint, causing a permanently swollen knee with poor mobility.

What Is the Treatment?

Surgery is the treatment of choice. The patellar groove is deepened to prevent the sideways (luxating) movement of the patella. Additionally, sutures are placed to hold the patella in a more normal position. Surgical correction generally has a good outcome, and the patients lead a fairly normal life.

ARTHRITIS (OSTEOARTHRITIS)

Osteoarthritis is generally referred to simply as arthritis. Osteoarthritis, technically speaking, is an inflammation of the bone structures of the joints. Although many things, such as injury or infections, can cause arthritis, most cases are simply due to aging. This discussion is about osteoarthritis due to the normal aging process.

As the patient ages, the normally smooth cartilage surfaces of the joints erode and wear thin. As this erosion takes place, it is repaired by the body, but the new surface is irregular. These rough surfaces of the joint then cause pain and additional inflammation when the bones articulate or meet with each other. The large joints, such as the shoulder, elbow, hip and ankle, are the most frequently involved; however, all joints, including those of the spine, can be affected. Obese patients tend to be affected the most, as the excess weight places a greater strain on these joints. Depending on the stress placed upon the joints, some days the pain is worse than others.

What Are the Symptoms?

Virtually every geriatric patient will have some degree of osteoarthritis; however, some will never exhibit symptoms. As in humans, stiffness, pain and swelling of the joint areas is commonly noted. The pain may be chronic or intermittent, mild or severe. Osteoarthritis is progressive, and the symptoms usually worsen with age.

What Are the Risks?

Osteoarthritis and its accompanying symptoms are not life threatening, but they do worsen throughout the animal's life. Many patients simply live within the limitations caused by the arthritis. Others with more severe pain may need some treatment to improve the quality of life.

What Is the Treatment?

In those patients experiencing pain, various anti-inflammatories have been used successfully. Overweight patients should be placed on a diet. Fortunately, most patients respond well to therapy, ensuring a quality life with minimal symptoms. Although aspirin is occasionally used to relieve pain in dogs suffering with arthritis, its use is not recommended for felines except under strict veterinary supervision. Cats have a very low tolerance to aspirin drugs when compared to dogs and humans. Aspirin, even in low doses, has been known to cause seizures in cats.

FRACTURES

Occasionally, due to abnormal stress placed upon the skeletal system, fractures or breaks of the bones may occur. Complex terminologies are used to describe all the possible fracture types and the proper correction of such. Basically, we refer to fractures not based on the name of the bone broken, but rather on the characteristics of the break itself. There are four commonly seen fractures in the feline (see figure 8-7): **closed, compound, epiphysial (growth plate)** and **greenstick (hairline).**

Closed fractures are those in which the skin is not broken; the bone is fractured, but the skin is intact. Conversely, **compound fractures** are breaks in which the broken bone protrudes through the skin and is exposed to the outside. Compound fractures are risky in that the bones are frequently contaminated with dirt and may become infected.

Epiphysial fractures are commonly seen in young, growing kittens. Bones grow from the ends. In animals less than one year of age, there are soft areas near the ends of each long bone where growth takes place. These soft areas are referred to as growth plates or epiphysial plates. Because these are areas of growth, they are rich in immature

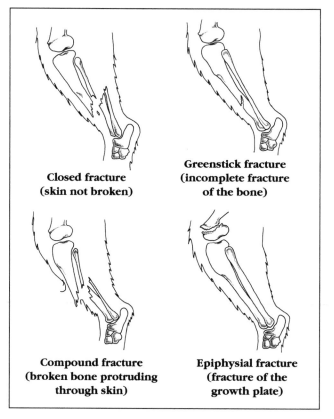

Closed fracture
(skin not broken)

Greenstick fracture
(incomplete fracture
of the bone)

Compound fracture
(broken bone protruding
through skin)

Epiphysial fracture
(fracture of the
growth plate)

8-7   Bone fractures

non-calcified cells that form a soft, spongy area of the bone. These growth plates are easily fractured because they are the weakest part of the bone. The distal ends of the femur and humerus seem to be particularly susceptible to this fracture.

Greenstick fractures are small cracks within the bone that leave the bone basically intact, but cracked. In other words, the bone is not completely broken.

What Are the Symptoms and Risks?
The symptoms and risks depend on the areas fractured and the severity of the fracture. Fractures involving a joint are more serious than those of other areas. A broken back, for example, may displace the spinal cord and cause paralysis. Typically, when a bone within a leg is broken, the cat will hold the leg off the ground. No weight is placed on the paw. With a sprain or lesser injury, it may use the leg somewhat, but walk with a limp. All fractures are serious and should be treated at once.

What Is the Treatment?

As with humans, splints, pins, steel plates and metal screws can all be used to realign the bone and promote proper healing. Growing patients may heal in as little as five weeks, while in the geriatric patient it may take twelve weeks or more for the same bone to heal. Hairline fractures may only require rest, while surgical intervention will usually be needed in more severe fractures. Cats, when compared to dogs, have a uniquely great ability to heal broken bones. Careful evaluation by a veterinarian will determine the proper treatment.

TUMORS OF THE BONES

Although rare, tumors of the bones do develop. Most are a malignant type called osteosarcoma. They are more common in geriatric patients than in younger animals.

What Are the Symptoms?

Usually, a notable swelling will be detected over the area of the tumor. In the early stages, however, there may be no symptoms. Most tumor sites are very painful on examination. The most common areas for bone tumors in the cat seem to be the sinuses and the long bones of the legs.

What Are the Risks?

Bone cancer is serious and life threatening. Most patients live less than one year; however, treatment may extend the life expectancy.

What Is the Treatment?

Treatment varies depending on the tumor location. If a limb is involved, then amputation may be required. Radiation and chemotherapy may also be used to treat some forms of cancer.

DISORDERS OF THE MUSCLES, LIGAMENTS AND TENDONS

Damage or malfunctioning of these organs is not as serious as injuries to the bone, but nevertheless they are commonly encountered and require proper treatment.

RUPTURED CRUCIATE LIGAMENT (KNEE JOINT)

Two cruciate ligaments, called the anterior and posterior ligaments, are found within the knee joint. Due to trauma, these can become torn or ruptured. In most damaging knee injuries, the anterior ligament is the one commonly ruptured. In more severe injuries, the posterior ligament will be torn as well. These two ligaments stabilize the knee joint by connecting the femur bone to the tibia. When these become ruptured, the two bones will move back and forth independently of each other, preventing the joint from functioning normally. This is referred to as a "drawer movement" because the movement is similar to the opening and closing of a drawer. Common causes of injury are slipping on icy or wet surfaces and automobile accidents.

What Are the Symptoms?

Initially the cat will limp, often severely, and may hold the leg off the ground and not use it at all. In time, the knee joint will become enlarged and fluid-filled. Any patient limping on the rear leg should be examined by a veterinarian.

What Are the Risks?

Without treatment, the patient will always limp or walk on only one rear leg. Consequently the unaffected rear limb will suffer undue stress and may also develop a ruptured cruciate ligament. In time, the affected knee will enlarge, scar and become immobile. The earlier the treatment is instituted, the more likely its success.

What Is the Treatment?

All cases of ruptured cruciate ligaments require surgery. Various surgical techniques are available to stabilize the knee by replacing the function of the torn ligaments. The ligaments are not repaired, but rather *replaced* either with synthetic material or tissue from other parts of the body. Surgery is very successful; however, the knee is generally not restored to 100 percent of its original mobility.

HERNIATED DISC (SLIPPED OR RUPTURED DISC)

As in humans, the feline vertebrae, which extend from the skull through the tail, are separated from one another by flexible cartilaginous discs (see figure 8-8). These discs provide a cushioning effect and permit the neck, spine and tail to bend, allowing changes in positioning and posture. Above the discs and running through the bony vertebrae is the spinal cord. The spinal cord extends from the brain and ends in the sacral area, near the base of the tail.

As the cartilaginous discs become weakened from age, disease or trauma, they may herniate or rupture. This causes portions of the disc to protrude upwards and place pressure upon the spinal cord. This

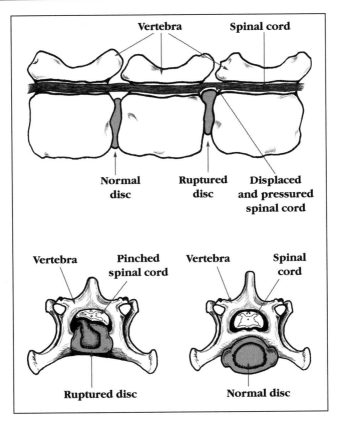

8-8   Normal and slipped disc

pressure may cause damage to the spinal cord and/or prevent nerve transmission through it. When a disc herniates, the damage to the cord may range from severe to very slight depending on the extent of the abnormal disc movement. Any injury to the spinal cord can result in pain, weakness or paralysis. Also, the location of the disc disease will affect the cord differently. A disc herniation in the neck (cervical) area will affect the body from the neck down. A herniated disc in the lower back (lumbar) area will only affect the rear limbs and loin or hip area. Severe cases affect the cat's control over urination and defecation as well.

What Are the Symptoms?
A herniated disc is intensely painful. Patients with herniation in the neck (cervical) area will hold the head lower than normal and will not want to flex it upwards or from side to side. They may have difficulty eating. A severe herniation in the neck area can cause enough damage to the cord to cause paralysis in all four limbs.

The most common disc herniation occurs in the lumbar (back) area. Generally these patients will hump their backs in response to the pain. In severe lumbar disc herniations, the rear limbs will be partially or completely paralyzed. Depending on the degree of damage to the cord, this may be temporary or permanent. Nerves to the anus and bladder may also be affected.

As you can see, the symptoms vary greatly depending on the location and extent of disc herniation.

What Are the Risks?

Injuries to the spinal cord are always serious. Complete or partial paralysis can result. The risk of long-term irreversible paralysis is greatly reduced if treatment begins at once, that is, within hours. Spinal injuries are an emergency.

What Is the Treatment?

Treatment always involves the use of anti-inflammatories, such as cortisones. These medications cause the herniated disc and swollen tissue to shrink and also relieve swelling and inflammation within the spinal cord. Surgery to remove the disc or surrounding bone is a viable option; it is best if surgery is performed within the first 24 hours following the injury. The recovery period may take from weeks to months. In severe disc herniations, a full or even partial recovery will not always be possible. The degree of recovery is never predicted, and only time will reveal the extent of a recovery.

Although various new anti-inflammatories have been approved for use in dogs, they have not been approved for cats.

C H A P T E R 9
The Nervous System

The nervous system is a complex network of electrical transmissions that functions similar to a computer. Electrical impulses travel through nerve fibers that deliver messages to, and control functions of, other cells and organs within the body. Chemical reactions also facilitate communication between nerve cells and the tissues.

The feline nervous system is divided into several segments. The **central nervous system (CNS)** is made up of the brain, brain stem and spinal cord (see figure 9-1). The **peripheral nervous system (PNS)** includes the nerves that run from the brain to areas of the head and neck, and also to nerves exiting and entering the spinal cord. These nerves carry messages from the CNS to other parts of the body. Nerve impulses travel from the brain down the spinal cord, out through the peripheral nerves, to the tissues and back again (see figure 9-2).

Peripheral nerves that go from the brain or spinal cord are called motor nerves because they affect muscles—they control movements, posture and reflexes. Peripheral nerves that return to the brain or spinal cord are referred to as sensory nerves because they carry information from the body's structures back to the central nervous system.

Another set of nerves that are part of the nervous system is the **autonomic nervous system (ANS).** The ANS (which comes from the CNS) contains nerves that control involuntary movements of organs such as the intestines, heart, blood vessels, bladder, etc.

HEAD TRAUMA

Trauma to the head can result from falling or, for example, being struck by an object. The main concern in cases of head trauma is injury to the brain.

What Are the Symptoms?

Symptoms vary depending on the severity of the damage. Different areas of the brain are responsible for different functions, so an injury to one area will affect the patient in one way, whereas injury to another area will probably have a completely different affect even in the same cat.

A wide range of symptoms can indicate injury to the brain. Nystagmus is a term used to describe rapid, uncontrolled eye movements. The eyes will appear similar to those of a person who is looking rapidly and repeatedly from side to side without moving the head. Anisocoria is a term used to describe a patient having one large pupil and one small pupil. In other words, the eyes are not functioning together. Pinpoint pupils or an extreme reduction in the size of the pupillary opening typically indicates a concussion of the brain.

Head tilt is another indicator that something may be wrong with the brain. If a feline receives injury to the left side of the brain, then the head may tilt to the left. Circling is yet another indicator of a brain injury. The pet will walk in small, tight circles and circle towards the injured side. In some cases, head tilt and circling will be seen simultaneously.

Seizures or convulsions are typically noted when the brain is damaged or irritated. In severe injuries, the patient may lie unconscious or be in a comatose state. In very mild injuries, however, there may be no noticeable signs. A headache in a cat would probably go unnoticed.

Regardless of the signs observed, symptoms rarely indicate the seriousness of the injury and do not relate to the probability of recovery.

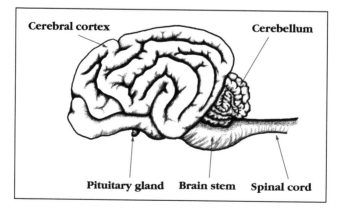

9-1   Feline brain, brain stem and spinal cord

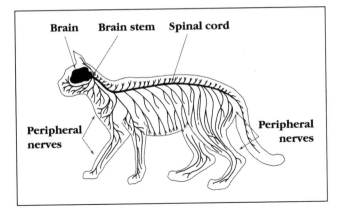

9-2 Feline nervous system

What Are the Risks?

Trauma to the brain is always serious. Damage to the brain tissue may be transient or permanent. Death can easily result if the condition is left untreated.

What Is the Treatment?

Always see your veterinarian at once if damage to the brain is suspected. Your veterinarian will administer drugs such as dexamethasone (an injectable steroid) and/or mannitol (an intravenously administered sugar solution that draws excess fluid from the central nervous system) to minimize brain swelling and inflammation. Rest is also important.

Generally, if brain damage occurs, the healing process will probably take weeks to months to complete. It is usually very difficult to predict the outcome when the patient is first examined, and in a few cases, it may take months before a veterinarian can predict if the patient will recover completely or to what extent recovery will take place.

TUMORS OF THE BRAIN AND SPINAL CORD

Tumors of the central nervous system are rare, but occasionally a patient is afflicted with brain cancer.

What Are the Symptoms?

The symptoms are much like those of a brain injury except they develop slowly and usually progress despite treatment. Typically, tumors of the brain or spinal cord are fatal. An accurate diagnosis can be made only from sophisticated tests, not clinical signs.

What Are the Risks?

In all cases, tumors of the brain and spinal cord are serious and life threatening. Early treatment should be sought.

HYDROCEPHALY

Hydrocephaly is a congenital condition in which excessive fluid is found in and around the brain. Within the brain are fluid filled spaces called ventricles (see figure 9-3). In a hydrocephalic patient, the ventricles contain too much fluid and become swollen. The increased pressure damages and/or prevents development of brain tissue. The body may form too much fluid, or as occurs in most cases, the fluid that is produced cannot drain from the central nervous system as it normally does.

What Are the Symptoms?

Generally the first symptoms appear when the patient is young, usually less than four months of age. The head takes on a dome-shaped appearance and the skull bones at the top of the head fail to close. This is termed "open fontanel" (see figure 9-4). The affected patient may have a soft spot on the top of the head, may be blind, have seizures or an altered gait. Different levels of severity exist.

What Are the Risks?

A patient with hydrocephaly will generally have a shortened life expectancy. Severity differs, but few cats live to be two years of age.

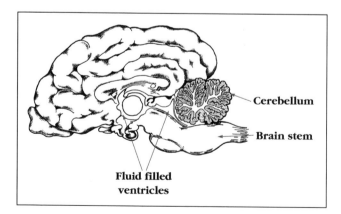

Cerebellum

Brain stem

Fluid filled
ventricles

9-3   Brain ventricles

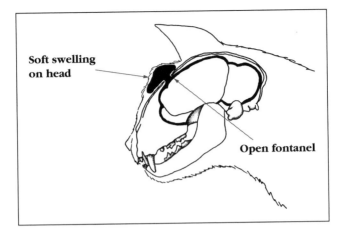

Soft swelling on head

Open fontanel

9-4   Open fontanel

What Is the Treatment?

Most cases go untreated. Veterinary neurologists can be consulted and occasionally the excess fluid can be drained. However, the patient rarely will live a normal life. Treatment is often unsuccessful and prohibitively expensive. *Hydrocephaly is a genetic/congenital disease and cats with this condition should be removed from any breeding program.*

SEIZURE DISORDERS (EPILEPSY)

Any insult to the brain such as trauma, infection or drug overdose can cause a seizure. Most seizures in the cat are not due to detectable causes such as trauma; however, most seizures are caused by idiopathic (unknown cause) epilepsy, a condition veterinarians generally refer to only as epilepsy. Detectable causes of seizures are those commonly associated with toxins, infections, drug overdose, trauma to the head area, and other metabolic disorders such as diabetes mellitus and kidney or liver failure.

The exact cause of epilepsy is not known, but whether the cause is unknown or trauma induced, the condition results in an uncoordinated firing of the neurons (nerves) within the brain. Normally, the neurons transmit impulses in a uniform and coordinated fashion, allowing for precisely timed movement and thoughts. During an epileptic seizure, however, the neurons function independently of each other. When the neurons misfire, patients may lose consciousness or become unaware of their surroundings, and have rapid, uncoordinated body movements.

Seizures may result from trauma, infections, and toxins. In some instances, they are inherited.

What Are the Symptoms?

Normally the epileptic patient will have the first seizure between two and three years of age. This time frame may vary, but rarely is epilepsy seen in the very young. Seizures will vary in intensity and are usually described using three terms: **petit mal, grand mal,** and **status epilepticus.**

Petit mal seizures are the mildest form. The patient may simply develop a blank stare, shake one leg or cry out in pain. Petite mal seizures usually last less than one minute. **Grand mal** seizures are the most common. This seizure is characterized by a patient falling to one side, urinating or defecating uncontrollably, paddling the feet as if swimming, frothing at the mouth and possibly crying out. This patient will be unaware of surrounding activities. Grand mal seizures usually last five minutes or less. **Status epilepticus** is the most severe form of seizure. It appears exactly like a grand mal seizure, but it may last for several hours. It may happen that as soon as recovery seems to occur, the patient immediately degenerates back into the seizure.

What Are the Risks?

Epilepsy is a chronic disorder and although usually not curable, it can be controlled. The petit and grand mal seizures, in most cases, are not life threatening unless they occur at a time when the feline is in an unsafe or uncontrolled environment.

Status epilepticus is a very serious seizure state. With the body convulsing violently for hours, the internal body temperature will become critically high. Organ damage and death can result. All seizure instances should be reported immediately to your veterinarian.

What Is the Treatment?

In most instances, epilepsy is not life threatening unless status epilepticus develops. Anticonvulsant medications are used in chronic cases. It must be understood that drug therapy does not cure the condition, but rather controls the severity and frequency of the seizures. Anticonvulsant drugs such as Phenobarbital may be used in the cat. Phenobarbital provides a sedative action on the nerves within the brain.

The goal of therapy is to stabilize the nerves and membranes within the brain, but not to a point where the patient appears or acts sedated. Generally, anticonvulsant drugs are not given unless the patient has more than one seizure per month or the seizures last more than half an hour. This is only a general guideline.

INFECTIONS OF THE BRAIN, THE SPINAL CORD AND RELATED STRUCTURES

Infections of the brain are called **encephalitis,** while those that involve the **spinal cord** are referred to as **myelitis.** A tough, protective layer of connective tissue called the *meninges* covers the central nervous system. An infection of this tissue is termed **meningitis.**

An infection of the central nervous system can involve any or all of these structures. Many different viruses and bacteria can enter the central nervous tissue and cause an infection. The most notable central nervous system diseases are rabies, feline infectious peritonitis (FIP), feline leukemia and toxoplasmosis. For a more complete discussion of these diseases, please see Chapter 15, "Common Feline Parasites" and Chapter 16, "Infectious Feline Diseases."

Bacterial infections may cause seizure disorders, although this is uncommon in the feline.

What Are the Symptoms?
Symptoms vary greatly, but may include fever, disorientation, confusion, blindness, staggering, vomiting, seizures and loss of consciousness.

What Are the Risks?
All central nervous tissue infections are serious. Death will likely result if the condition is left untreated. If an infection is suspected, call a veterinarian at once.

What Is the Treatment?
With any central nervous system infection, the affected tissue is irritated and swollen. Since these tissues are encased within the skull and back bones, as the nervous tissue expands, individual cells are damaged or destroyed as they are crushed against the surrounding bone. This can result in irreversible damage.

In cases of central nervous system infection, much of the therapy is aimed at controlling the swelling of the tissues. Intravenous solutions, such as mannitol or corticosteroids, are used. Mannitol is a diuretic that helps remove excess fluid, therefore reducing swelling around the nervous tissue. Corticosteroids reduce inflammation and pain associated with tissue damage. Whenever a bacterial infection is present, high levels of antibiotics are used. There are no specific medications that can eliminate or destroy viruses. With the exception of rabies, viruses must be allowed to run their course.

The patient will be supported with intravenous fluids, often nourished through feeding tubes and protected from fluctuations in body temperature. Because of the risk to humans, from rabies and other organisms causing infections of the central nervous system, treatment must always be weighed against the probability of cure and the risk of infection to others.

MOTION SICKNESS

Cats, as well as humans, may suffer from motion sickness. The vast majority of suffering from motion sickness arises as the result of travel in a motor vehicle. The exact cause of motion sickness is unknown, but the detection of movement both by the visual and vestibular systems plays a role.

What Are the Symptoms?
Most cats suffering from motion sickness will initially salivate profusely. The eyes are usually dilated. As the illness progresses, the cat will vomit and may develop diarrhea. Unique to the cat, compared to a dog or human, is the fact that when stressed, a cat can shed hair in immense quantities. This may accompany the gastric upsets.

What Are the Risks?
Although the cat appears violently ill and stressed, motion sickness is neither life threatening nor permanent. More serious conditions, such as epilepsy or cardiac disorders, however, may worsen as a result of the stress associated with motion sickness.

What Is the Treatment?
Although not always preventable, there are measures one can take to help reduce the incidence and severity of motion sickness.

It is best if the cat is not fed for several hours before the trip. As a conditioning exercise, take the cat on frequent, short (15-minute) rides in a slow-moving vehicle. This will acclimate the cat to transportation and help accustom it to more lengthy trips. While traveling, most cats will feel more secure in a covered crate or carrier designed for travel. This helps eliminate the visual triggering of motion sickness.

Tranquilizers and antihistamines will help some patients that are extremely sensitive to the effects of travel. These are obtainable through veterinarians.

CEREBELLAR HYPOPLASIA

The area of the brain responsible for coordination is the *cerebellum* (see figure 9-5). Occasionally the cerebellum will fail to fully develop and remain smaller than normal, hence the condition referred to as cerebellar hypoplasia. Despite common belief, there is no scientific evidence to suggest that this condition is inherited. The cause is due to an infection of the unborn fetus by a parvovirus called feline panleukopenia, which is commonly known as feline distemper. If the mother is exposed to this virus while pregnant, the virus can cross into the placenta and affect the development of the fetal brain. It is also possible for cerebellar hypoplasia to be the result of a mother being vaccinated against feline distemper while pregnant.

What Are the Symptoms?
The cerebellum is largely responsible for the coordination of voluntary movements such as walking. The affected kitten will usually develop a lack of coordination by eight weeks of age. It will have difficulty walking and eating, and will suffer tremors and vibrate (shake) while attempting to move. At rest, it will usually appear normal. Weight loss will result following the inability to eat adequate amounts of food.

What Are the Risks?
A kitten with cerebellar hypoplasia will become critically ill as it grows. Death will result before the kitten reaches maturity and usually will occur much sooner.

What Is the Treatment?
There is no treatment for cerebellar hypoplasia. Once identified, most owners opt for euthanasia to prevent the eventual death due to starvation.

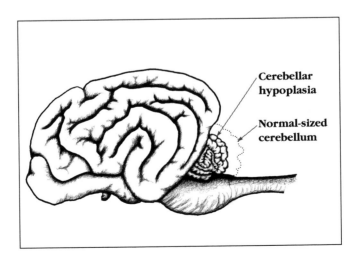

9-5 Feline cerebellar hypoplasia

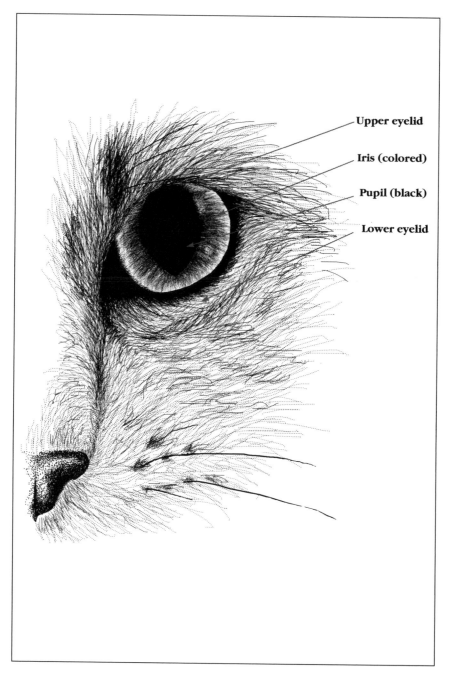

Upper eyelid

Iris (colored)

Pupil (black)

Lower eyelid

10-1   Feline eye

The Eye, Eyelids and Surrounding Tissue

For centuries, humans have been intrigued and fascinated with the cat's large eyes and steady gaze.

And indeed, the eyes are a cat's most important sensory organ. Compared to other mammals, such as humans and canines, a cat's eyeballs are extremely large in proportion to the head (see figure 10-1). Perhaps because the cat's other senses, such as smell and hearing, are not as extensive as those of some other mammals, the cat has evolved to utilize sight as the primary organ of sensory detection. A hunter by nature, the cat's large eyes with their wide peripheral vision serve as the principal tool for detecting prey.

The eyeball is an organ that processes light. Once the light enters the eyeball, the cells within the eye convert the light to electrical impulses that travel through the optic nerve to the brain. The brain interprets them, thus creating images (see figure 10-2).

The eye is protected by being sealed in a strong, bony eye socket supported by tissues of lubrication, muscles and eyelids. Additionally, the back of the eyeball rests against a cushion of soft fatty tissue that provides some protection against excess pressures placed against the eye.

The eyeball is formed by several layers of tissue. The unpigmented portion or "white part," called the **sclera,** is made of tough fibrous tissue rich in blood vessels, which transports oxygen and nutrients to the eye structure. The **cornea** is the transparent or "window-like" outer portion of the eyeball. The cornea has several layers of uniquely arranged cells that make it transparent. Light passes through the cornea, thus enabling the cat to see. Inside the eyeball are specialized structures suspended in a liquid called **vitreous fluid.** These fluids provide nutrients and oxygen to these inner eye structures; they also put pressure on the interior

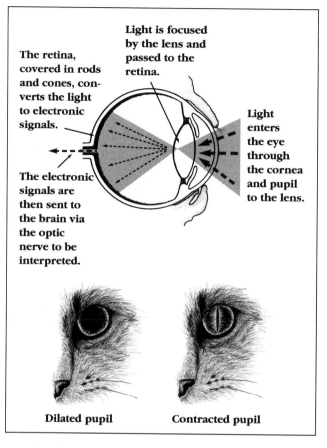

The retina, covered in rods and cones, converts the light to electronic signals.

Light is focused by the lens and passed to the retina.

Light enters the eye through the cornea and pupil to the lens.

The electronic signals are then sent to the brain via the optic nerve to be interpreted.

Dilated pupil   Contracted pupil

10-2   The eye and its functions

of the eyeball, thus keeping it inflated, maintaining its "ball-like" shape (see figure 10-3).

The colored portion of the interior eye is the **iris.** In humans, the iris may be different colors. The majority of cats possess green or yellow eyes, but other colors such as blue and copper exist, particularly in certain breeds. It is not unusual for a cat to have two different color irises, for example one blue eye and one green eye. The color of the iris, coupled with the largeness of the eye, certainly adds to the beauty of the feline.

The opening through the iris is the **pupil.** In contrast to the circular pupil of the human and the canine, the feline pupil is elliptical, being longer than it is wide. The opening or size of the pupil can be made larger or smaller by muscles called ciliary bodies that attach to the colored iris, causing it to expand or contract. In dim light the pupil is made larger or wider, enabling more light to enter the eye. Conversely, in bright conditions, the pupil becomes narrower, almost

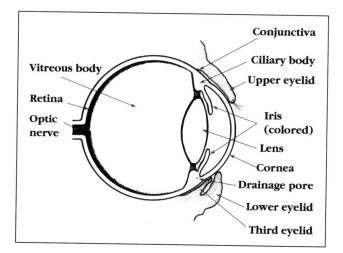

10-3   Components of the feline eye

slit-like. This is important because too much light can cause pain and even damage the inner structures of the eye.

Behind the pupil lies the **lens,** a pea-sized organ resembling a marble, which is normally clear. The lens is suspended by tiny ligaments, which hold it directly in the center of the eyeball so that light will pass through it. The lens bends, concentrates and focuses light rays that enter the eye and pass through the pupil. Once focused by the lens, the light rays pass to the rear surface of the eyeball, called the retina.

The **retina** contains nerve cells referred to as *rods* and *cones.* The rods are sensitive to the intensities of light, while the cones help detect color. Unlike humans, the feline possesses very few cones, therefore *cats are colorblind.* Like the dog, it is believed the domestic cat only sees white, black and shades of gray. Although they cannot see colors like humans do, cats possess a visual capability that we do not have. The retina in most cats is rich in reflective cells, forming a mirror-like structure called the tapetum lucidum. In very dim light conditions, such as nighttime, the light rays striking the tapetum lucidum are reflected and intensified, enabling the cat to have night vision. This creates the characteristic greenish-yellow reflection when light is shone upon it. Odd as it may seem, not all cats are created equal in this sense. Some cats, most notably those of the Siamese breed, lack the greenish-colored pigmentation of the retina. Despite the difference in reflectivity, the Siamese do appear to have adequate night vision. When light shines into the eye, the retina reflects red rather than greenish-yellow.

As previously stated, nerve cells within the retina transform light energy into nerve impulses. The nerve impulses are concentrated and exit the eyeball via the **optic nerve,** where they are carried to the brain. The brain then translates the impulses into images, creating vision.

The eyeball is surrounded by a soft, pinkish tissue called the **conjunctiva.** The conjunctiva connects the eyelids to the eyeball. The feline, like the dog, has three eyelids in contrast to the human, who has only two. The lids of the feline are called the upper, lower and nictitating membrane (see figure 10-4). The nictitating membrane is usually referred to simply as the third eyelid. The third eyelid plays important roles in the production of tears, and contains lymphoid tissue that helps prevent infections of the eye. To view the third eyelid, simply apply slight pressure to the eyeball with your finger (see figure 10-5). The third eyelid passively moves from the nasal corner to partially cover the eye.

When a cat is tired or resting contentedly, the third eyelid will generally partially obscure the eyeball. Although not a true indicator of health, the ailing feline may also carry the third eyelid partially closed. Such is the case of the dehydrated or excessively thirsty cat whose eyeball has sunk abnormally into the socket. All three lids and surrounding structures contain lubricating tarsal and lacrimal glands that produce a fluid called tears to bathe and flush the eye. The upper lids also contain eyelashes that help prevent dirt and other particles from

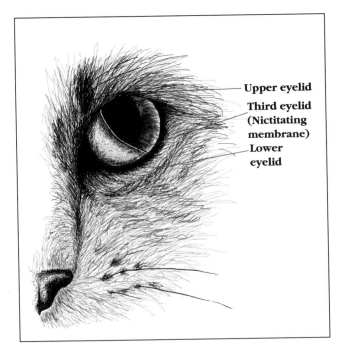

10-4   Eyelids of the feline

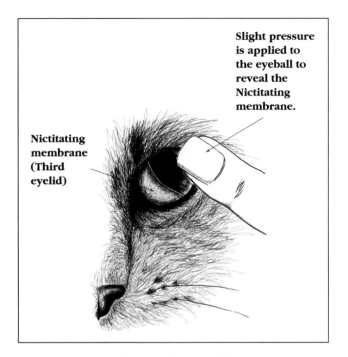

10-5   Nictitating membrane or third eyelid of the feline

falling upon the cornea. Tears provide moisture to the eye and help flush out dust, pollens and other fine debris that might otherwise irritate the eye.

The three eyelids and surrounding conjunctiva work to lubricate, nourish and protect the eyeball. The **tear glands** supply the tears that flush and cleanse the eye surface. Tears exit the eye and its related structures through a small duct or opening at the inside corner of each eye. These ducts, one for each eye, are called the lacrimal or tear ducts (see figure 10-6). Tears also help prevent eye infections because they kill many kinds of bacteria entering the eye. Disorders of these tissues usually create a very reddened eye, frequently with excessive or altered tear production (hence the term "red, runny eyes.") In reality the eyeball may be perfectly fine, but the tissues around the eye are irritated and inflamed. This often is referred to as *conjunctivitis* if the conjuntiva is involved. Because of its large size and exposure to the elements, ailments of the feline eye and its surrounding tissues are common.

CONJUNCTIVITIS

The pink, membranous tissue surrounding the eye and attaching to the eyeball is the conjunctiva. When this tissue is inflamed, the cat is

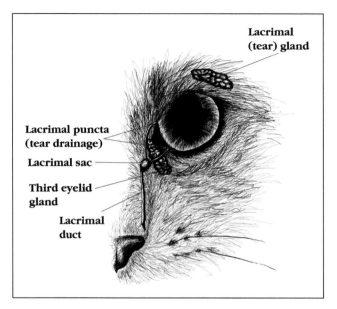

10-6 Lacrimal system of the feline

said to have a conjunctivitis. The conjunctiva may be inflamed due to allergies to substances such as dust, pollens, weeds, smoke, etc. In the cat, bacterial and viral infections of the conjunctiva are not uncommon. The best-known bacterial cause is due to the organism *Chlamydia psittaci,* commonly referred to as psittacosis or parrot fever. The two best-known viruses that affect the conjunctiva are calicivirus and rhinotracheitis virus. (For a more in-depth discussion of these three infectious diseases, please refer to Chapter 16, "Infectious Feline Diseases.")

If the white portion of the eyeball, known as the sclera, is also inflamed and pink, the condition may be referred to as *"pink eye."*

Conjunctivitis is the most common ailment affecting the eye structures of the cat.

What Are the Symptoms?
Commonly, both allergies and infections will cause a reddened or meaty appearance of the conjunctiva. In both cases there may be an increase in fluid about the eye, causing the eye to "run." The characteristics of the discharging fluids can help determine the cause. With irritations due to *allergies,* the eye discharge is generally clear, as the glands surrounding the eye are simply producing more tears to help flush away the allergens. This is the same type of discharge a human may experience while peeling an onion.

Infections generally cause the eyes to produce a thick, yellow-to-greenish fluid. The eyes become crusty and may even stick shut when closed. Infections stimulate the body to produce white blood cells to fight off the invading organisms, and it is the white blood cells that give the eye discharge its thick and yellow consistency. Some people refer to this as a "mattering of the eye." We usually use the term "matter" to describe the normal accumulation of fluid and crust about the eye, especially while sleeping. A small amount of matter is expected to develop in every cat and is not indicative of a disease.

Any irritation around the eye, whether infectious or not, will likely cause the cat to squint, thus allowing the third eyelid to cover the nasal portion of the eye. Additionally, the cat may paw the area around the affected eye in an attempt to soothe the area, much as humans would rub their own eyes.

What Are the Risks?

Normally, a conjunctivitis is not life threatening unless the organisms travel to the deeper structures of the eye. In the cat, however, it is important to determine the cause. Infectious diseases such as chlamydia, rhinotracheitis and calicivirus may affect other organs such as the lungs (see Chapter 16, "Infectious Feline Diseases"), as well as the conjunctiva. These diseases can advance and cause severe illness or even death. Kittens in particular are at the greatest risk for severe eye trauma. Infections can also spread to other individuals. In fact, chlamydia can even spread from cats to humans as well as other cats.

Allergies are not life threatening and are commonly present throughout the cat's life. Allergies are not contagious, and therefore pose no threat to other cats or humans. Persians, with their compressed faces, commonly have misalignment of the lids and/or an incomplete lid closure, making them one of the most susceptible breeds to develop a conjunctivitis.

What Is the Treatment?

Conjunctivitis should be treated at once and, if possible, the cause identified. In the case of a bacterial conjunctivitis, antibiotics, applied either orally or directly onto the eye tissues, are usually curative. If allergies are the suspected cause, then eye drops or ointments containing an anti-inflammatory such as hydrocortisone are usually used. The treatment length varies depending on the cause, but usually the minimum time is seven days. Vaccines are available to prevent the diseases Chlamydia, rhinotracheitis and calicivirus. These are usually administered to all cats, even house cats, on an annual basis.

MEIBOMIAN GLAND INFECTIONS

The meibomian glands are small glands laying in a line on the inner surface of the upper and lower eyelids. Their primary function is to secrete an oily lubricating substance that upon blinking is spread over the eyeball surface to keep it moist. These small glands open to the inner lid surface through microscopic pores. Bacteria sometimes enter these pores and cause an infection to develop inside the lid margins. Occasionally, cysts develop. Frequently this occurs as a result of a bacterial conjunctivitis that has gone untreated, therefore progressing to advanced stages.

What Are the Symptoms?
The eyelids become smaller, red and very painful. Frequently a yellow discharge will be noted, causing the entire eye to appear sticky and crusted.

What Are the Risks?
An infection of the lids and their associated meibomian glands is extremely uncomfortable. The cat will rub at the eyes in an attempt to alleviate the pain. In acute or untreated cases, the lids will severely abscess and portions may actually die and slough tissue.

What Is the Treatment?
Every case of eyelid infection should be treated at once. A culture may be necessary to identify the bacteria so the appropriate antibiotic can be

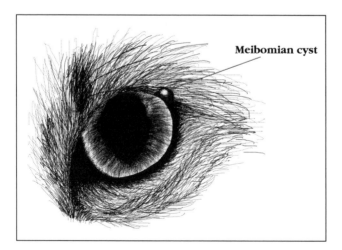

10-7   Meibomian cyst

selected. Oral antibiotics as well as antibiotic ointments are typically administered simultaneously for periods of up to several weeks or until recovery is complete. Cysts may require surgery.

ENTROPION

This is a condition in which the lower lid margins roll inward to the extent that hair rubs on the surface of the eyeball (see figure 10-8). All breeds may be affected; however, it is more common in Persians and shorter-faced cats than others, suggesting it's an inherited trait.

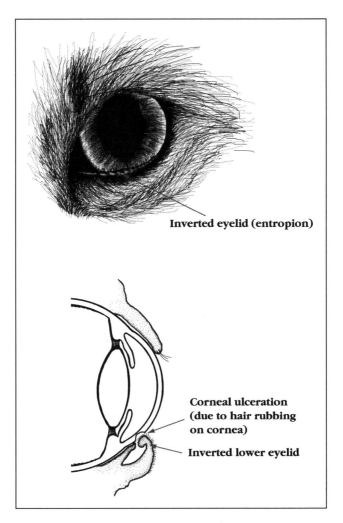

Inverted eyelid (entropion)

Corneal ulceration (due to hair rubbing on cornea)

Inverted lower eyelid

10-8 Entropion feline eye

What Are the Symptoms?

A cat suffering with entropion will generally squint and have chronically reddened eyes. Because of the abrasive effects of an abnormal hair touching the cornea, the corneal surface may erode, causing a corneal ulceration as a secondary effect. In chronic cases left untreated, the corneal surface will become scarred and pigmented. Occasionally, an ulcer will perforate the cornea, allowing bacteria to enter the inner eye structures, usually resulting in blindness.

What Are the Risks?

Blindness, or at best a severely scarred cornea with impaired vision, will be the result of chronic, untreated cases. Since most cats that develop this condition are born with it, it's best to start treatment at an early age, usually around four months.

What Is the Treatment?

Surgery is the treatment of choice to correct the abnormal lid. Usually, a small elliptical incision is made below the lid that when sutured, pulls the lid outward to "unroll" it. This prevents the hair from abnormally touching the corneal surface. With surgery, a complete recovery is expected.

ECTROPION

Ectropion describes a condition in which the lower eyelid is loose and sags downward (see figure 10-9). It is the opposite of entropion described above. Although common in canines, it is rarely found in felines.

What Are the Symptoms?

With the sagging of the lower lid, the membranes (conjunctiva) surrounding the eyeball are exposed, forming a pocket-like pouch. This area commonly collects dust, pollens, bits of grass, etc., all of which irritate the conjunctiva, causing it to appear reddened. It is a painful condition that provides opportunity for infection.

What Are the Risks?

The risks are not great and many patients live a normal life. In severe cases in which the area becomes chronically inflamed, treatment is recommended.

What Is the Treatment?

Surgery is the treatment of choice. The area lateral to the lower lid is incised and "tucked," thus tightening the lid. Once the lid is tightened,

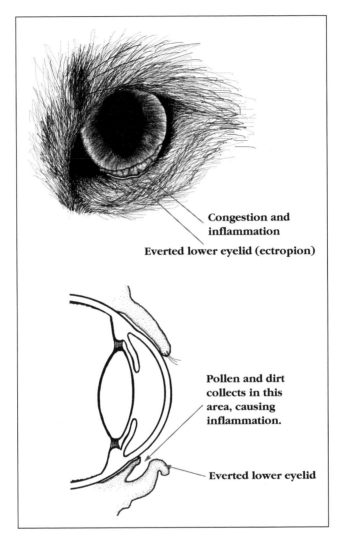

Congestion and
inflammation

Everted lower eyelid (ectropion)

Pollen and dirt
collects in this
area, causing
inflammation.

Everted lower eyelid

10-9   Ectropion feline eye

or pulled laterally, the conjunctiva is no longer abnormally exposed. A
full recovery is expected.

EVERTED THIRD EYELID

Occasionally the third eyelid or nictitating membrane will fold over on
itself. This is termed an **eversion.** It happens only to the third eyelid,
not the upper and lower lids. Although this condition is present spo-
radically in all breeds, Burmese have a higher occurrence, which
suggests an inherited condition in that breed. The third eyelid contains
a small supporting cartilage that may be defective, thus allowing the

folding to occur. While folded, the third eyelid cannot move and provide proper lubrication for the eye. Infections of the eye, specifically the cornea, may be the result.

What Are the Risks?
Commonly the everted or folded third eyelid poses an opportunity for infection. Because of the largeness of the feline eye, proper lubrication is necessary. Occasionally with an everted third eyelid, there may be an inadequate lid closure, resulting in inadequate lubrication.

What Is the Treatment?
A third eyelid eversion is corrected surgically. The defective cartilage is partially or completely removed, thus allowing the lid to unfold back into its normal position. It is very important not to remove the lid or its glandular structures, as they play a principal role in lubricating the eye surface.

FOREIGN BODIES BEHIND THE THIRD EYELID

The third eyelid moves upward over the cornea from the bottom of the eyeball nearest the nose. Because the third eyelid is a flap, it is not uncommon for foreign materials (foreign bodies) such as dust, small sticks, hair, bits of straw, weeds and the like to lodge under the third eyelid. When this happens, the third eyelid cannot move properly. When it does close, the offending material is moved over the cornea and the abrasive effects can cause damage.

What Are the Symptoms?
Usually the foreign material is small enough that it is not easily detected under the third eyelid. One simply notices the cat is squinting as if the eye is painful. Additionally, the cat may paw about the eye as a result of the discomfort. The eye will tear more than normal.

What Are the Risks?
Typically, if the foreign body is not promptly removed, it will irritate the cornea, and an ulcer will form. A corneal ulcer is always serious and in this case will worsen until the offending material is removed. The ulcer may puncture the cornea and result in blindness.

What Is the Treatment?
Foreign bodies under the third lid are not easily found. Only careful observation will reveal their presence. A topical anesthesia may be needed to "freeze" the eye, allowing one to grasp and view behind the third eyelid. Usually with the aid of a topical anesthetic and a small

forceps (tweezers), the bits of foreign material can be removed. Once the foreign body is removed, antibiotic eye preparations may be necessary to prevent infections and allow any corneal ulcers or abrasions to heal.

PROMINENT NASAL FOLDS

Nasal folds arising from the muzzle immediately below the eye may be so pronounced that they rub on the cornea. Brachycephalic cats (those with compressed faces, such as Persians and Himalayans) are most likely to be affected (see figure 10-10).

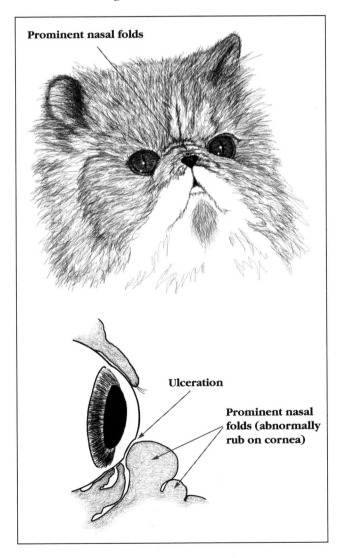

10-10   Prominent nasal folds

What Are the Symptoms?

Usually the patient will have excessively runny eyes. The folds covered with hair have an abrasive effect upon the eye surface, thus providing the source of irritation. A simple visual examination will reveal the prominent folds and hair rubbing against the corneal surface.

What Are the Risks?

The abrasive effect of the hair upon the cornea is both discomforting and destructive. It is not uncommon for ulcerations to develop upon the corneal surface. These are always serious.

What Is the Treatment?

Treatment involves surgery to remove or decrease the size of the nasal fold. Early treatment is best to prevent damage to the cornea. It is expected that the prominent folds would be completely corrected by surgery.

PLUGGED LACRIMAL DUCT

Tears and lubricating oils produced by the various glands around the eye all have a common drainage. A small but visible pore is found on the lower lid near the nose. This is the **lacrimal puncta** and is the opening into the tube-like tear duct (also referred to as the **lacrimal duct**). The lacrimal duct drains tears from the eye margins into the nasal cavity. It is not uncommon for the tear duct to become plugged, thus preventing the normal drainage of tears. It may become plugged as a result of excess dust and debris, but more commonly it is the result of infections within the duct itself. Once bacteria enter the duct, they may inflame the duct walls. When the duct walls become thickened, the opening may swell shut. Due to infections, a thick, yellow discharge may develop about the eye, especially near the nasal surface.

What Are the Symptoms?

Patients with plugged lacrimal ducts will appear to have an excessively watery eye. In reality, the tear production is normal, but since drainage is impeded, tears build up, spill over the lower lid and drain down the face from the inside corner of the eye. This usually discolors the hair with a dark brown streak. If the duct or eye is infected by bacteria, a thick yellow discharge may appear within the eye.

What Are the Risks?

For the eye to be properly lubricated, the ducts need to function correctly. If the ducts are plugged, this is uncomfortable but certainly not life threatening. Rather, the eye is more prone to infection, and the hair becomes discolored. In some cases the chronic, moist exudate causes the skin below the eye to become irritated. Bacteria can invade and clog these ducts and cause severe and painful infections. If this is suspected, treatment should begin at once.

What Is the Treatment?

The lacrimal duct is "re-opened" by flushing out the restrictive material. A small needle is placed into the opening of the duct and saline is flushed downward (through the end of the nose), providing cleansing action. Anesthetic may be required. If an infection is suspected, then oral antibiotics and eye drops are used as follow-up treatment. This problem may occur in animals with abnormal or thicker tear secretions, or in cases where the duct is abnormally formed or has been damaged.

EPIPHORA—TEAR STAINING

In some cats, especially Persians and Himalayans, tears drain down the face from the nasal side of the eye (see figure 10-11). The problem is generally thought of as one of excessive tear production. This is not the case at all as tear production is normal in these individuals. The cause is improper tear drainage. This may be the result of plugged tear ducts and/or an abnormal nasal structure that prevents tears from entering the duct. When tear drainage is impeded, the tears simply spill down over the face. Once on the facial hairs, the tears react chemically with skin bacteria and create a pink to brown stain on the hair or form a crust. Additionally, the hair under the eye may mat.

What Are the Symptoms?

The main symptom is simply a pink to brown stain on the facial hair below the nasal side of the eye. In light-colored cats, the stain is more pronounced. A crust may develop immediately under the eye.

What Are the Risks?

The main risk is infection, if the hair becomes matted and/or a thick crust develops. Frequently when the crusted mat is removed by hair trimming, the skin immediately under the mat is found to be inflamed or even infected. Being moist and mat-covered, this area creates a perfect environment for bacteria to grow.

What Is the Treatment?

If a plugged tear duct is suspected then it may be necessary to flush it open. If bacteria are suspected, antibiotics should be administered. It

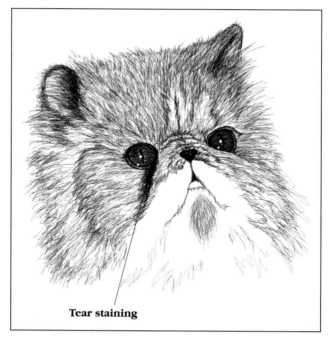

Tear staining

10-11   Tear staining

should be noted that in the authors' experience, 97 percent of all cases of tear staining are not due to infections or plugged tear ducts; the cause is simply an abnormal configuration of the lower lid drainage area. Persian and Himalayan breeds are most susceptible, and tear staining in these instances is not really the result of a medical condition, but rather facial structure. Commercially prepared tear-stain removers are available to minimize the effects of staining. Hair susceptible to matting should be trimmed regularly. In an attempt to prevent the chemical reaction from taking place, antibiotics such as Tetracycline are sometimes used to help decrease facial bacteria. This is of questionable value and is generally not the recommendation of the authors. Most cases require no treatment whatsoever. Simple cleanliness and grooming are all that is necessary to maintain health.

RETROBULBAR ABSCESS

Occasionally pockets of infection (abscesses) will develop behind the eyeball. Usually only one eye is involved. Although the cause is difficult to determine, it is suspected that bacteria enter through the mouth and gum line and cause a pocket of infection to become trapped behind the eyeball. Cats that eat chicken bones are at the highest risk as these bones frequently splinter and can easily poke through the skin.

What Are the Symptoms?

Retrobulbar abscesses usually cause the eyeball to protrude or bulge from the socket. The eye may be repositioned at a strange angle, causing the affected eye to be "looking off to the side." Almost always, the patient will experience pain when the mouth is opened. When the animal attempts to eat or drink, the jaw bone places increased pressure behind the eye. If an abscess is present within that area, severe pain may result. Most patients will stop eating as a result of the pain.

What Are the Risks?

Any suspected cases should be treated at once. Not only are the pain and discomfort a concern, but any infection this close to the eye and its nerves can easily spread throughout the eye.

What Is the Treatment?

Surgical drainage of the abscess is the quickest and surest way to treat the condition. An incision is made inside the mouth immediately behind the last molar. Once the abscess is drained, the patient will recover quickly. Following surgery, oral antibiotics are used to treat the bacteria.

DISORDERS OF THE EYEBALL

Compared to relative body size, the eyeball of the domestic feline is one of the largest of all mammals. It is ironic that cats' eyes, which give them so much mystique, are also their vulnerability. Because of the large, exposed surface area, feline eyes are particularly susceptible to injury and disease.

The eyeball is made of several structures including the **cornea, colored iris, lens, anterior and posterior chambers** and the **retina** (see figure 10-12). The three lids—*the upper, lower* and *nictitating membrane (third eyelid)*—lubricate and protect the eyeball. Additionally, the eyeballs are partially protected by bony ridges surrounding the eye socket within the skull. Trauma, infections and metabolic disorders can all affect the health of the eyes.

FOREIGN BODIES IN THE CORNEA

Any abnormal objects within the body are referred to as foreign bodies. The front portion of the eyeball, or cornea, is particularly exposed

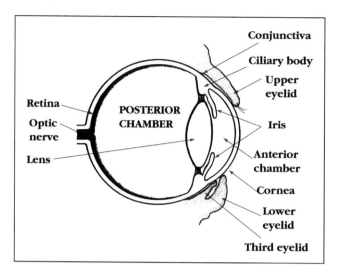

10-12   Components of the feline eye

and subject to injury. Foreign bodies such as sticks, seeds, weeds and dirt frequently cause damage to and/or become lodged in the cornea. The foreign body can be visible or may be hidden behind the lids, most commonly under the third eyelid. In these cases, as the animal blinks, the material will move and cause an abrasion on the cornea.

What Are the Symptoms?
Most patients with a foreign body injury will experience some pain. They tend to squint or blink excessively. They may rub the eye either with a forepaw or slide the entire head across the carpet in an effort to remove the offending material. This causes further damage.

What Are the Risks?
The cornea is a delicate, easily damaged structure. Abrasion can lead to a corneal ulcer. This in itself requires treatment, but the problem may not stop there. Loss of vision is a real possibility if the cornea is severely damaged and especially if it is punctured. A puncture allows bacteria or other organisms to gain access to the inside of the eyeball.

What Is the Treatment?
If the foreign body is lodged in the eye, it must be removed immediately. Flushing with warm water or saline may wash away the particles. More severely lodged foreign bodies, such as sticks or splinters, may require surgical removal. Antibiotic ointments are usually applied to

minimize infections. It is important to examine behind the third eyelid for foreign material. This is a common place for bits of weeds or seeds to be hidden from view. No eye exam is complete without examining behind the third eyelid.

ULCERS OF THE CORNEA

The cornea or transparent portion of the eye is made up of several layers of cells uniquely arranged so as to be transparent to light. This is why the front portion of the eyeball is clear, thus enabling the cat to see through it. Any erosion of the cell layers making up the cornea is termed an ulcer, specifically a corneal ulcer (see figure 10-13). Ulcers generally develop as a result of trauma or infections of the cornea.

CORNEAL ULCERS CAUSED BY INFECTIONS

HERPES VIRUS INFECTIONS

An inflammation of the cornea by a herpes virus is referred to as a **herpetic keratitis.** Usually cats over six months of age are the most susceptible; young kittens are not at much risk.

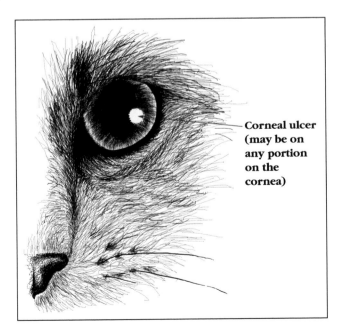

Corneal ulcer (may be on any portion on the cornea)

10-13 Corneal ulcer

What Are the Symptoms?

The most noted sign of a cat suffering from a herpetic keratitis is a cornea that appears hazy, often with an ulcer large enough to be noted with the naked eye. The herpetic ulcer may be small, linear or branching. A branching ulcer is considered diagnostic for a herpes viral infection.

What Are the Risks?

The ulcers may be minor or severe depending on the individual patient's immune capability of fighting viral infections. In severe cases the cornea will become severely scarred, greatly impeding vision.

What Is the Treatment?

Corneal ulcers caused by a herpes virus pose a medical challenge because they are difficult to cure. Some success has been achieved with various anti-viral drugs such as Idoxuridine (IDU) and Trifluoride. Used in both ointment and droplet form, they are placed directly into the infected eye. Various steroidal preparations (hydrocortisone) have also been used with some success in combination with anti-viral drugs. Steroids should not be used alone as they can make the condition worse.

CORNEAL SEQUESTRATION

Corneal sequestration is used to describe a situation in which the cornea and its cells simply degenerate. Persians, Himalayans and Siamese cats have the highest incidence of this condition. This implies that genetics plays a role, at least in these breeds. There is no known cause.

What Are the Symptoms?

Usually both eyes are affected. As the layers of the cornea die, they slough off and form an ulcer. Some authorities refer to this as a "melting of the cornea." The area also develops visible blood vessels with deposits of black or brown pigment found directly on the cornea.

What Are the Risks?

As the cornea degenerates, it is very possible for an ulcer to perforate the cornea and expose the inner eye contents. This can result in blindness in the affected eye(s).

What Is the Treatment?

Although the cause is unknown, the condition in the early stages usually responds favorably to antibiotics and topical steroids. Occasionally, surgery to repair the corneal ulcer may be beneficial. In general, the condition can be controlled, but not cured. Treatment is aimed at reducing the possibility of a corneal perforation and loss of vision.

TRAUMA TO THE CORNEA

Of the domestic animals, felines have the highest incidence of trauma to the cornea. As discussed earlier, this is due to their disproportionately large, prominent eyes. Cats also love to play, sometimes in rough fashion. This coupled with sharp claws oftentimes leads to scratches of the eyeball. Damage to the cornea as a result of physical injury is commonly encountered.

What Are the Symptoms?
Scratches or other corneal trauma are initially very painful. The patient may squint the eyelids and paw the area in an attempt to alleviate the discomfort. Tear production will usually be dramatically increased as the body tries to "flush out" the irritation. The third eyelid often moves up over the cornea, partially covering it. The actual scratches or bruised area may or may not be visible upon initial examination. Specialized instruments such as ophthalmoscopes may be required to make an actual diagnosis. Specialized fluorescein dyes can be added to the eye to highlight or outline the area of damage. This is generally done in a hospital.

What Are the Risks?
Any trauma to the cornea has the potential to be serious. Deep scratches may permeate the cornea and cause blindness. Most minor scratches, although initially very painful, will eventually heal. Total healing time may be two weeks to a month or more, depending on the extent of damage to the cornea.

What Is the Treatment?
The most common treatment is the application of antibiotic eye drops or ointment to prevent bacterial infections from developing. Later in the healing process, eye medications containing steroids may be applied to minimize scarring of the otherwise transparent cornea. In severe injury cases, surgery may be performed to close the third eyelid so as to cover the damaged area while it is healing. This technique is referred to as a "third eyelid flap." The eye is only temporarily closed, usually for a period of three to five days. Other similar types of surgery may be performed in specialized cases. Always have a veterinarian examine the patient if trauma to the eyeball is suspected. With early, vigorous

treatment, a full recovery can be expected. In untreated and severe cases, blindness may result.

HEREDITARY CORNEAL DYSTROPHY

Hereditary corneal dystrophy is most often seen in the stump-tailed cats of the Manx breed. It is generally seen in older kittens about four to six months of age. In corneal dystrophy, various elements including calcium and fats are abnormally deposited within the cell layers of the cornea. Over a period of several years, the normal cells of the cornea begin to degenerate and die. Both eyes will eventually become diseased.

What Are the Symptoms?
The cornea will initially appear normal, but as the disease progresses will become hazy and "bluish." As the cells of the cornea become infiltrated and die, fluid builds up within them. This is referred to as edema, more specifically corneal edema. The edema and fatty deposits result in the bluish cast of the normally transparent cornea.

What Are the Risks?
As corneal dystrophy progresses, the cells of the cornea die and eventually erode away. A rupture and destruction of the cornea results in blindness. Blindness in both eyes usually occurs by the time the patient reaches middle age.

What Is the Treatment?
There is no treatment for corneal dystrophy. It is thought to be an autosomal, recessive gene. *Affected individuals should not be bred.* Through genetic selection the incidence of the disease can be reduced, despite the fact it is not treatable.

DISORDERS OF THE EYE CHAMBERS

The eyeball is a hollow structure incompletely divided by the iris into the anterior and posterior chambers (refer to figure 10-12). Both chambers are filled with vitreous fluid, which bathes and nourishes the inner eye structures. Vitreous fluid is produced within the eyeball and drains outward into the veins. Since the amount of vitreous fluid production precisely equals what drains out, a consistent shape and fluid pressure within the eyeball is maintained.

GLAUCOMA

Glaucoma is a term used to describe increased pressure within the eye. When vitreous production exceeds drainage, fluid builds up within the eye, causing increased pressure. Glaucoma may be of the primary or secondary nature. Primary glaucoma is not caused by another unrelated condition. There is simply too much vitreous fluid, either from an excess production or decreased drainage. Secondary glaucoma is an increased pressure due to other eye disorders such as lens luxation. In either case, one or both eyes may be involved.

What Are the Symptoms?

Regardless of cause, a patient suffering with glaucoma will have a swollen and very painful eye. The pupil will be large (dilated) and unresponsive to light (see figure 10-14). In other words, it will not constrict even when a bright light is shined directly into the eye. Squinting is common and the pain may be so great as to cause depression and a lack of appetite. The animal will often rub its eye against the carpet or furniture. The cornea may appear bluish, and the white portion of the eye will be reddened with enlarged blood vessels.

What Are the Risks?

All cases of glaucoma are medical emergencies. As the pressure builds within the eye, blood vessels, nerves and other structures within the eye become damaged and blindness results.

What Is the Treatment?

Eye pressure is measured with a veterinary device called a tonometer. The exact extent of increased pressure is determined and the proper

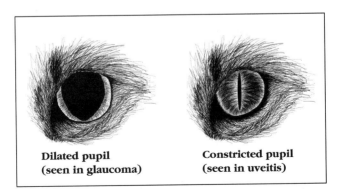

Dilated pupil   **Constricted pupil**
(seen in glaucoma)   **(seen in uveitis)**

10-14   Dilated and constricted pupils of the feline

treatment is selected. Therapy is aimed at decreasing vitreous production and increasing vitreous drainage, thus decreasing and stabilizing the inner eye pressure. Veterinarians use a variety of drugs, such as Pilocarpine and Daranide, to accomplish this. Surgery may be indicated in cases of primary or secondary glaucoma.

UVEITIS

Uveitis is an inflammation of the anterior chamber of the eye including the iris and ciliary body (tissue supporting the lens). Bacteria and fungus are often the cause. They may enter the eye through the bloodstream or by an injury to the cornea or other eyeball surface.

What Are the Symptoms?
Uveitis causes the eye to become shrunken and soft, just the opposite of glaucoma. The patient will squint, usually with excess tearing. Whereas patients with glaucoma have unusually large pupils (dilated), patients with uveitis have unusually small, or constricted pupils (see figure 10-14). Pain is severe. Usually only one eye is involved.

What Are the Risks?
All cases of uveitis are medical emergencies. Left untreated, blindness is the end result.

What Is the Treatment?
Cortisones are used in many cases to fight inflammation. Atropine is administered to dilate the pupil. If an infection is present, then antibiotic and/or antifungal drugs may be prescribed in addition to the above. Proper treatment requires the examination and care of a veterinarian.

DISORDERS OF THE IRIS

The colored structure of the eye is the iris. By expanding or contracting, the opening through the iris, called the pupil, regulates the amount of light entering the eye. In bright light, the cat has a small "slit-like" opening, while in dim light the pupil takes on a more rounded appearance.

IRIS CYSTS

Occasionally the iris may develop small, round, dark spots that are not firmly attached. These are iris cysts. The cause is unknown and generally no treatment is used, as they do not affect the iris's function.

ALBINISM

Occasionally one or both irises of a cat may not be pigmented. This is usually seen in all-white or predominately white cats. The iris may be multi-colored or pink and may be accompanied by deafness in the ear on that side. Albinism is not really a disease, but rather a genetic trait. No treatment is necessary.

PERSISTENT PUPILLARY MEMBRANE

The **iris** continues to develop in the newborn up to two weeks of age. In a newborn kitten, the iris is a single piece of tissue, lacking the opening called the **pupil.** Beginning just prior to birth and continuing for about two weeks, the cells making up the center of the iris die and create an opening forming the pupil. None of these changes are recognizable to the owner as the kitten's eyelids remain closed at least until about two weeks of age. Occasionally when the pupil is forming, the tissue that dies will persist as small fibrous strands. These are known as persistent pupillary membranes.

What Are the Symptoms?
With some tissue persisting, the hole that becomes the pupil is irregularly shaped and is crisscrossed by fibrous strands (see figure 10-15).

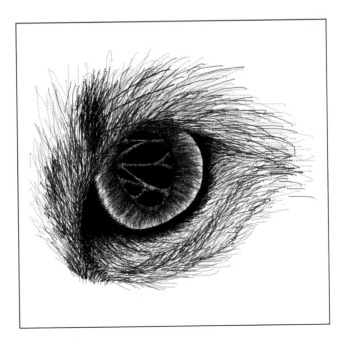

10-15 Persistent pupillary membrane

The pupil, rather than being an elliptical opening, may give the appearance of a black, glass marble with cracks coursing through it.

What Are the Risks?

Cats with persistent pupillary membranes generally live normal lives. If the pupil is unable to expand or contract properly, however, they may be shy of certain light intensities. This would probably go unnoticed to the owner and would pose no threat to the health of the cat.

What Is the Treatment?

There is no medical treatment for persistent pupillary membrane. In unique instances surgery may be attempted to remove excessive tissue adhesions. This procedure is rarely recommended or necessary.

DISORDERS OF THE RETINA

The very back of the eyeball is the retina. The retina is a membranous structure composed of cell layers. This cellular membrane transforms light into electrical impulses that are transmitted by the optic nerve to the brain where "vision" is created. Any disorder of the retina may drastically affect the patient's ability to have normal vision.

DETACHED RETINA

The layer of cells known as the retina may on occasion become separated or "detached" from the eyeball capsule. This may be the result of trauma or another disease. Diseases such as **f**eline **i**nfectious **p**eritonitis (FIP) (see Chapter 16), cancer and high blood pressure may secondarily affect the retina and cause it to detach from its connective surface.

What Are the Symptoms?

A partially detached retina may go unnoticed by the owner. If the detachment is complete, a loss of vision in the affected eye will be evident.

What Are the Risks?

A detached retina poses a severe threat to the patient's vision. The detachment may be partial, initially progressing over time to a complete detachment and consequent vision loss. It is extremely important to carefully examine the patient and identify the reason for the detachment. More severe life-threatening disorders may be an underlying cause.

What Is the Treatment?

Treatment depends on identifying the cause and treating it and the retinal detachment concurrently. Medications, such as the steroid Prednisone and the diuretic Lasix, are used to reduce inflammation and fluid accumulation, allowing the retina to reattach. Mild cases may heal with no medical intervention. Treatment is oftentimes successful if more serious underlying diseases are not present.

TAURINE DEFICIENCY

Taurine is an essential amino acid in the cat. Most cat foods and feline nutritional supplements are fortified with taurine to help prevent deficiencies. Cats suffering from deficiencies of taurine are usually being fed inadequate diets. Cats fed foods designed for dogs are most likely to suffer from this—taurine is not necessary in the diet of the canine, so dog foods usually contain extremely low levels of this amino acid.

What Are the Symptoms?

A cat suffering from a taurine deficiency will eventually suffer from a loss of vision due to degeneration of the retina. *Additionally, serious, even life-threatening disorders of the heart will arise.*

What Are the Risks?

A taurine deficiency is always serious. Blindness and/or loss of life due to cardiac abnormalities may result.

What Is the Treatment?

Once identified, the taurine dietary deficiency must be corrected. Once adequate levels of taurine are ingested by the cat, the degeneration of the retina cells is usually stopped. It is important to note that the damage incurred by the retina and heart may be permanent, but further damage will be prevented by proper nutrition. Dog foods and non-meat–based diets are inadequate for the nutritional maintenance of the feline. Lesions on the retina, from diets low in taurine, begin to develop in cats fed inadequate amounts for four months or more. An occasional meal of an improper diet will not harm the cat.

DISORDERS OF THE LENS

The small marble-like structure located immediately behind the pupil is the lens. Small fibers that attach it to the inner surfaces of the eyeball suspend it in the proper position. By altering the lens shape, the eye can focus on objects and project these "in-focus" images to the retina. The normal lens is transparent, so disorders of the lens commonly alter the transparency and cause blurred vision.

LENS LUXATION

If the small fibers that hold the lens in place weaken, the lens is no longer secured and it moves from its normal position behind the pupil (see figure 10-16). The fibers securing the lens can also be damaged as a result of head trauma. One or both eyes may be affected.

What Are the Symptoms?

Usually, as the lens slips from its normal position, vision is disrupted. This is a problem, but the greatest danger of a luxation of the lens is that it may block drainage of the inner eye, or vitreous fluid. When fluid accumulates within the eye, increased intraocular pressure occurs. This extremely painful condition is referred to as glaucoma. (See page 151.)

What Are the Risks?

Lens luxation affects a patient's vision, but *if glaucoma develops and goes untreated, blindness will almost certainly result.*

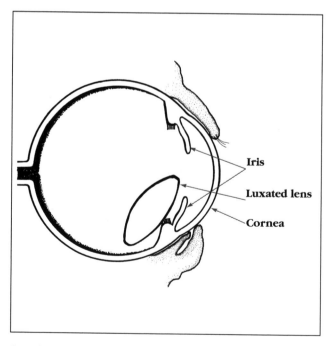

10-16 Lens luxation

What Is the Treatment?

Generally surgery is recommended to remove the entire lens. Once the lens is removed, vision is impaired, but present.

CATARACTS

The normal marble-like lens is approximately 66 percent water and 34 percent protein. If this delicate balance of water to protein is altered, cataracts can form. Excess levels of protein cause deposits that create small, dense areas within the normally clear lens. These are termed cataracts. A patient with cataracts will not have a clear lens; instead it will appear cloudy and often with an internal latticework of lines similar to that seen in ice cubes. There are several types of cataracts; one type is routinely seen in patients suffering with the disease affecting blood sugar levels, diabetes mellitus.

JUVENILE CATARACTS

Juvenile cataracts develop while the patient is still a kitten, that is, less than one year of age. Although this type of cataract is not common in kittens, it may be detected in kittens at two months of age or younger. Genetics may be a factor as Persians, Himalayans and Birmans are most commonly affected. Typically, both eyes are affected, although occasionally just one eye will develop this disease.

ADULT CATARACTS

Adult cataracts develop as the feline ages, with most patients being middle-aged or older when the cataracts are first noticed. Some texts refer to adult cataracts as senile cataracts; however, the authors do not prefer this term as it implies senility or extreme age. Adult cataracts typically develop after six years of age. They generally appear as small, white areas within the lens. If the cataracts are not severe, they may not deter vision. In severe cases, blindness will result if the condition is not treated.

DIABETIC CATARACTS

As in humans, pets with diabetes mellitus often develop cataracts. In this instance, the abnormally elevated blood sugar will cause sugar deposits to occur within the lens. This high concentration of sugar attracts excess fluid, which in turn causes a breakdown of cell membranes. The resulting protein deposits form cataracts.

What Are the Symptoms?

Regardless of the cause, various cataracts can appear quite similar. Other than the age and medical history, there is no easy way to determine the cause or type of the cataract.

Most cataracts are clearly visible to the naked eye. When viewing a patient from the front, one may notice small, white to milky-gray lines or areas throughout the lens. In more severe instances, the patient may have a vision defect serious enough to cause it to bump into objects. Mild or early-stage cataracts may not be visible without the aid of an ophthalmoscope used by an experienced veterinarian.

What Are the Risks?

The risks vary with the cause. Both juvenile and diabetic cataracts may progress to the point of causing blindness. Adult cataracts tend to develop slowly, and in some instances pose no real threat to the animal's vision. Juvenile cataracts develop more rapidly and at a much earlier age and are therefore likely to seriously impair vision. Abnormalities in these areas should always be referred to your veterinarian as soon as they are noted.

What Is the Treatment?

Once the cause or type of cataract has been identified, the appropriate therapy can be selected. In severe instances, cataract surgery, in which case the entire lens is removed, may be an option. Vision will be present, but impaired. Diabetic cataracts are very difficult to resolve. Correcting the blood sugar with insulin may help discourage further cataract development, but it will not affect changes that have already occurred. Most adult cataracts require no treatment as they tend to progress slowly. It is not recommended to breed animals with a known history of juvenile cataracts. Obviously, the issue of cataracts and treatment is a complex subject. Once a thorough understanding between the veterinarian and pet owner has been developed, the patient can be evaluated and the proper treatment selected.

NUCLEAR SCLEROSIS

This is a normal ocular change associated with aging. As one grows older, the lens, which is normally clear, takes on a hazy appearance. The majority of geriatric cats will have some degree of nuclear sclerosis.

What Are the Symptoms?

When we look straight into the feline's pupil, a hazy or blue-gray color will be seen. In severe cases, the feline may have difficulty seeing small objects at rest, but can usually detect motion. In most cases, vision will be only slightly affected and objects will appear as if one is looking through a dirty window.

What Are the Risks?
There is little risk to the patient. With age, nuclear sclerosis will progress; however, it rarely affects vision severely.

What Is the Treatment?
Usually treatment is not necessary in nuclear sclerosis. Removal of the lens would be possible, but is not warranted.

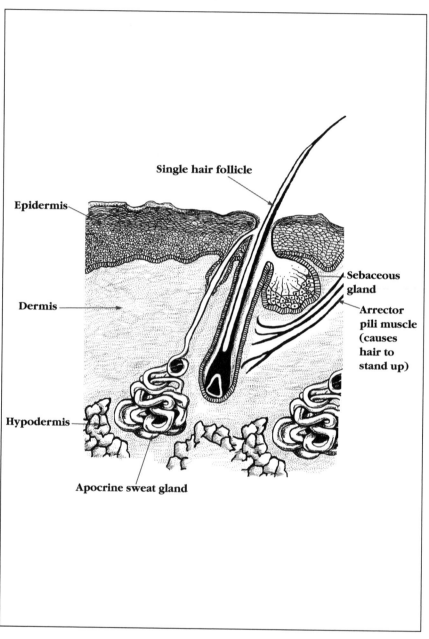

Single hair follicle

Epidermis

Sebaceous gland

Arrector pili muscle (causes hair to stand up)

Dermis

Hypodermis

Apocrine sweat gland

11-1   Cross section of skin

CHAPTER 11

The Skin, Hair and Nails

The skin, the body's largest organ, serves as a barrier between the cat and the outside world. It protects the cat from infections, parasites and the elements. It also maintains the body's internal environment by preventing loss of moisture and other body constituents. Because the skin is on the outside of the body, and therefore exposed, it is easily accessible to injury and disease. It is also very visible, so disorders are readily detected upon examination.

The skin is an organ made of layers of **cells, lubricating (sebaceous) glands, hair** and their **follicles, blood vessels** and **nerve endings.** The skin cells form layers, namely the tough outer covering called the *epidermis* and the deeper inner layer called the *dermis.*

The **epidermis** is composed of older cells that form a tough, almost impervious, protective outer barrier. As these cells erode, other cells mature and move upward to replace them. The epidermis is *thicker* on the more exposed areas, such as the head and back, and *thinner* in other areas, such as the armpits and belly.

The deeper layer, the **dermis,** contains hair follicles, blood vessels, nerves and sebaceous (oil) glands. Hair follicles and sebaceous glands are more prevalent on the back than on the belly. Most cats have two types of hair: a long, stiff outer coat and a short, soft, thinner layer for insulation. The hair coat and the variations between skin layers are dependent upon breed and climate. Both hair and nails are formed from dead cells hardened with keratin.

Although diseases of the skin, hair and nails are usually not life threatening, they can cause considerable discomfort and be unsightly.

STUD TAIL (FELINE TAIL GLAND HYPERPLASIA)

The top surface of the feline tail has an area rich in glandular tissue located about two inches out from the body. This area of the tail is sometimes referred to as the supracaudal organ. The glands of this organ secrete wax and oils to lubricate the hair around the tail and rump area. Occasionally the glands multiply and enlarge (hyperplasia); they secrete oils and wax in excessive amounts, often causing severe matting and even loss of hair immediately over and around this area. *Both male and female cats may develop this problem;* however, it is much more common in unneutered males. Because of the high incidence among unneutered males, it is often referred to as "stud tail."

What Are the Symptoms?

The most common symptoms associated with tail gland hyperplasia are excessive oils, matting and hair loss around the gland area. Occasionally there will be a complete hair loss over the gland. The gland may enlarge and appear raised and reddened.

What Are the Risks?

Tail gland hyperplasia from a medical standpoint is not serious. The gland may appear large and unsightly, but unless it becomes infected with bacteria, it is not painful. Bacterial infections of the gland are rare.

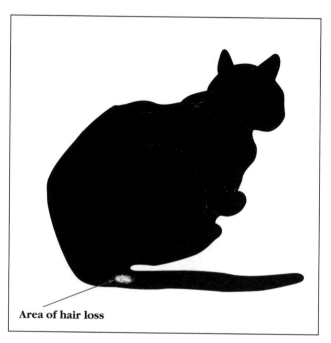

Area of hair loss

11-2   Stud tail

What Is the Treatment?

Treatment is aimed at managing the symptoms, not curing the disorder. Even with treatment, the condition will not go away. Benzoyl peroxide shampoos are excellent at cleansing the area. This helps remove excessive oils and odors, and reduces the incidence of infections associated with the gland. Hydrocortisone sprays will help eliminate inflammations of the cells. Neutering will usually help slow the progression of the disorder, but will not eliminate it. It is best if the area is simply cleansed daily with benzoyl peroxide shampoo. Excessive mats, if present, should be removed. Exercise and sunlight may also help reduce the progression. Sunlight probably dries the area, while exercise helps prevent excessive licking of the area, which may cause irritation.

IDIOPATHIC MILIARY DERMATITIS

Miliary dermatitis refers to a scabby skin irritation usually about the head, neck, back and rump area. Miliary lesions are small scabs about the size of a match head. Many affected animals have hundreds of such scabs, primarily over the back. *Idiopathic* means "of unknown origin." Idiopathic miliary dermatitis then refers to multiple small scab lesions without a known cause. It must be noted that other types of miliary dermatitis exist in which the cause is known. Examples include flea bite dermatitis, allergies and staphylococcus bacterial infections. Idiopathic miliary dermatitis can affect all cats; however, the authors are of the opinion that it is more prevalent in cats with black or gray coat colors.

What Are the Symptoms?

Cats with a miliary dermatitis will have multiple (often hundreds) small, scabby lesions over the head, neck, back and rump. The cat is usually otherwise healthy.

What Are the Risks?

In advanced cases, the patient may be severely itchy. Hair loss may be prevalent if the patient grooms excessively or scratches about the affected areas.

What Is the Treatment?

As mentioned, *it is absolutely essential to differentiate idiopathic miliary dermatitis, from other similar conditions.* Only when other cases of a dermatitis, such as allergies, parasites (fleas, lice, mange mites), fatty acid deficiencies, etc., are eliminated can the diagnosis of idiopathic miliary dermatitis be made. Once identified, idiopathic miliary dermatitis is responsive to drug therapy. Oral progesterone drugs such as megestrol acetate (Ovaban and Megace) have been used very successfully to treat this condition. Most patients respond favorably, although low-level treatment may occasionally be needed for extended periods of time throughout the life of the patient.

RINGWORM

Please see Chapter 16, "Infectious Feline Diseases."

FELINE ENDOCRINE ALOPECIA

Please see Chapter 7, "Hormone Disorders."

NEURODERMATITIS (PSYCHOGENIC ALOPECIA)

Neurodermatitis is characterized by a loss of hair due to excessive licking and grooming. Neurodermatitis is not a medical problem, but rather a psychogenic state of mind. Exactly why individual cats develop this problem is unknown. Excessive grooming to the point of hair loss may be similar to a human chewing fingernails. Neither is necessary, but seem to arise out of habit. In both cases, stress and/or boredom may be a triggering factor. It is more common in nervous cats than those that are calm by nature. Abyssinians, Siamese and Burmese have the highest incidence.

What Are the Symptoms?
The physical act of excessive licking or grooming may not be noticeable. The hair loss will be more apparent. Some cats only lick one small area, but most with this condition lick all body regions that are easily accessible. Many cats lick their belly, back and thigh areas. Normally the skin in these areas appears normal, but the hair is shortened, giving a shaved appearance.

What Are the Risks?
This is not a serious disorder; however, an occasional cat will lick and not only destroy the hair, but irritate the skin as well. Cosmetically, the cat will appear abnormal, as patches of hair will be missing.

What Is the Treatment?
It is important to determine if the cat is bored or stressed. Has it been confined to a small area? Have more cats been added to the household? Occasionally increasing exercise to reduce boredom will be beneficial. Various calming drugs such as phenobarbital, valium and megestrol acetate have been successfully used to treat this condition.

FLEA HYPERSENSITIVITY
(FLEA BITE DERMATITIS OR FLEA ALLERGY)

Many cats have fleas, but only a small majority have a hypersensitive reaction to the flea bite, more specifically the flea saliva. Despite the fact that only a small percentage of flea-infested cats have a hypersensitivity to fleas, a flea bite dermatitis is the most common allergy in the cat. In a cat not sensitive to flea saliva, the flea bite may cause only some minor skin irritation; the cat may not scratch at all, and the area bitten will appear normal. In cats with a flea hypersensitivity, however, the flea bite will set off a series of allergic reactions in the skin. The area will become intensely inflamed (reddened), followed by a severe itching. This is a result of the flea saliva initiating a hypersensitivity (or allergic) reaction in the skin.

What Are the Symptoms?

A cat with a flea hypersensitivity will itch and therefore scratch, especially about the head, neck and back area, although the whole body may be involved. The skin will become pink and irritated. Scabs may form over the affected areas. Secondly, bacteria may invade the damaged skin and cause oozing scabs to form. Hair loss, occasionally extensive, will be evident.

In most cases, fleas or flea feces (flea dirt) will be evident. It must be noted that as few as one flea bite per week can cause an allergic reaction. Just because fleas cannot be found does not mean that they are not present in small numbers. Remember, fleas do not live on pets, they merely feed there. At any given time they may not actually be present on the pet. For a more complete discussion on fleas refer to Chapter 15, "Common Feline Parasites."

What Are the Risks?

A cat suffering with flea allergies is miserable and may be so preoccupied with scratching that it loses weight because it has lost interest in food. Bacteria often invade the damaged skin and cause serious skin infections. Fleas also carry other diseases, such as tapeworm.

What Is the Treatment?

Once this condition is diagnosed, it is important that strict flea control measures be taken. The patient and the environment must be treated to eliminate and kill the fleas. To help with the allergic response, anti-inflammatories such as cortisones (Prednisone and Depo-Medrol™) are administered. This stops the inflammation and itching until the fleas can be eliminated.

SOLAR DERMATITIS

Solar dermatitis is a skin disorder of the nasal area, eyelids and ear margins resulting from repeated exposure to sunlight. Cats in the southern regions are most likely to be affected because as one nears the equator the sun rays become more intense. White cats are particularly susceptible because they lack skin pigment that helps block the effects of sunlight. A solar dermatitis is usually worse in the summer than in the winter months.

What Are the Symptoms?

The most common signs are scratching and inflammation of the affected regions. Hair loss and itching will occur in advanced cases. The nose, eyelids and ear flaps may be affected, but the ear flap margins are the most common areas to develop lesions.

What Are the Risks?

It is not uncommon for a solar dermatitis to cause severe ulceration on the affected areas. Skin cancer may also develop as a result of the repeated exposure to sunlight.

What Is the Treatment?

Affected cats should be isolated from direct exposure to sunlight. If this is impossible, topical sunscreens are partially effective at blocking the sunlight. Amputation of the ear flaps is warranted in severe cases.

SKIN CANCER

It is not uncommon to diagnose skin cancer in the cat. Various tumors are often referred to simply as "lumps," which develop from the deeper cells making up the layers of skin.

Squamous cell carcinoma is the most common feline skin cancer seen by the authors. This is usually seen about the head area, frequently on the nose, lips and eyelids. Most patients are six years of age or older. White cats have a higher incidence than others, probably due to lighter skin pigmentation. As in humans, sunlight may play a role in triggering the development of squamous cell carcinomas. *This cancer is malignant and often spreads to other areas of the body.*

Basal cell tumors are the second most common feline skin cancer seen by the authors. This tumor is found anywhere on the body, but most frequently on the top of the head and neck areas. Most patients are middle-aged and older when this cancer develops. Despite the fact that these tumors are frequently large, most are benign and are not serious.

Occasionally, the lubricating glands (cerumen glands) in the ears become cancerous. The ear canal is rich in these glandular structures; this is the area where the tumors develop. Most cats with this cancer are older, and usually only one ear is involved. *These tumors may be benign or malignant.*

Fibrosarcomas are malignant tumors that arise from the cells comprising the skin layers. A patient may simultaneously develop one or several of these tumors. Unlike most other skin cancers, fibrosarcomas are frequently seen in kittens as well as older cats. *This type of tumor can be serious if left untreated.*

The treatment of skin cancer in the cat usually involves surgery to remove the tumor(s). Once the tumor(s) is removed, it can be biopsied to determine the exact type of cancer and whether it is malignant or benign. Depending on the biopsy results there may be no further treatment after the surgery. Occasionally, anti-cancer drugs or radiation therapy is used.

With any form of skin cancer it is best if exposure by the cat to sunlight is limited.

FACIAL ALOPECIA

Alopecia is a term used to describe a baldness. It is not uncommon for older cats to experience a permanent thinning of the hair about the head.

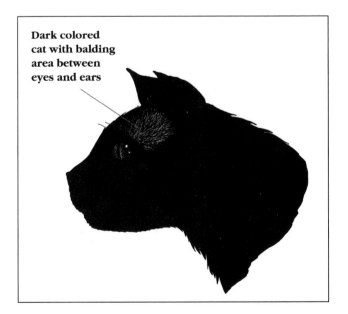

Dark colored cat with balding area between eyes and ears

11-3   Facial alopecia

What Are the Symptoms?

The most common area of normal hair thinning is between the eye and the ear (see figure 11-3). The hair loss will be symmetrical affecting both sides of the head. Although facial alopecia is common in all cats, it is most notable in those with dark hair. This is simply a result of the light skin contrasting with the darker hair.

What Are the Risks?

There is no risk associated with facial alopecia. It is normal and to be expected in middle-aged cats.

What Is the Treatment?

There is no treatment for facial alopecia.

ALLERGIC DERMATITIS

By definition, if an animal has inflamed and itchy skin, it probably has an allergy to something. Cats may be allergic to pollens, grasses, fleas and other insects, plastics, cigarette smoke, medications, carpet fibers, mites, detergents, food and many other things. Some allergies are due to things the pet inhales. Pollens and smoke fit this category and are termed "inhalation allergies." If the allergy is due to something ingested, we call it a "food allergy." Allergies due to carpet fibers, grass and plastics are termed "contact allergies." Those due to fleas are referred to as "flea allergies" or "flea bite dermatitis."

Whatever the allergy source, the principles are the same. The item the pet is allergic to is called the allergen. Allergens stimulate histamine release from within cells, which in turn causes the patient's skin to itch excessively. Scratching and chewing the itchy area is the hallmark sign of an allergy.

Depending on the cause, allergy flare-ups may be short-term, seasonal, or year-round. Seasonal allergies are the most common and are worse in the summer and fall when grasses and weeds produce the most pollen. This is also true in humans with hay fever, which is really a pollen or grass allergy. The average feline does not develop allergies until about three years of age; however, some younger patients are occasionally seen with them.

Although rarely life threatening, allergies can often make the patient miserable. A pet with allergies will be preoccupied with the itching sensation and will not be happy. Additionally, their coat and skin appearance will be poor and may produce an offensive odor.

What Are the Symptoms?

As previously mentioned, most patients with allergies suffer from extensively itchy skin. The skin may also be pink and inflamed, to the point of hair loss and bleeding. The areas most commonly affected will be the feet, the sides of the body and, in the case of flea bite dermatitis, over the back in front of the tail. These animals will also have frequent ear infections. With food allergies, the patient may also vomit or suffer from diarrhea.

What Are the Risks?

The main problem allergies present is that they are almost always a chronic source of some discomfort, usually itching. Allergies are controllable but seldom curable.

What Is the Treatment?

The treatment is dependent on the severity. Occasionally, veterinary dermatologists can perform allergy tests to identify the cause, and, through injections, they can hyposensitize the patient. Allergy testing, although useful, is expensive and not always successful. From a practical standpoint the allergic condition should be considered manageable, not curable. It's much like hay fever in people. Antihistamines such as Benadryl can be useful. In more severe cases, veterinarians may use potent anti-inflammatories such as cortisones to alleviate the itching and provide comfort for the patient.

Medicated shampoos with ingredients such as oatmeal and hydrocortisone are an aid for the patient with mild allergies. They will not eliminate all signs, but help in the overall treatment. Changing the diet may be beneficial in food allergies; however, food allergies are infrequently encountered. In instances of flea or mange mite allergies, it is very important to practice strict parasite control.

It must be understood by both owner and veterinarian that usually the exact cause of the allergy will not be determined. Treatment is aimed at controlling the allergic response, not necessarily finding a cure. Improving the quality of life for the allergic patient is the primary goal of therapy.

FELINE ACNE

Feline acne can affect cats of any age. The lesions typically develop just under the lower jaw (chin) and may spread along the lower lips (see figure 11-4). The cause is unknown, but frequently bacteria invade the area and irritate the hair follicles.

What Are the Symptoms?

A reddened and often crusty area will develop immediately under the chin. Large bumps or boils may develop. These are actually inflamed and occasionally infected hair follicles. In mild cases, "blackheads" will

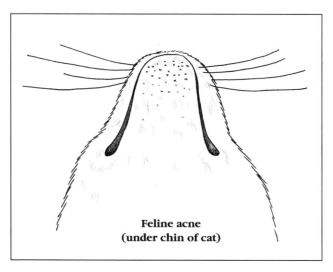

Feline acne
(under chin of cat)

11-4 Feline acne

develop and the chin simply appears dirty and crusty rather than inflamed.

What Are the Risks?

Feline acne is not really a serious disorder, but occasionally funguses (ringworm) and bacteria can invade the inflamed area and cause discomfort or pain.

What Is the Treatment?

The best treatment is to clean the affected area daily with a benzoyl peroxide shampoo. This cleanses and flushes the follicles. Antibiotics are used if bacteria appear to be present. Various anti-inflammatory drugs such as Ovaban (megestrol acetate) and cortisones are occasionally used in stubborn cases.

SCABIES

Please see Chapter 15, "Common Feline Parasites."

CHEYLETIELLA

Please see Chapter 15, "Common Feline Parasites."

LICE (PEDICULOSIS)

Please see Chapter 15, "Common Feline Parasites."

CUTEREBRA FLY LARVA

Please see Chapter 15, "Common Feline Parasites."

FLY STRIKE

Please see Chapter 15, "Common Feline Parasites."

EOSINOPHILIC GRANULOMA COMPLEX

Occasionally, cats develop bright red lesions on their skin or inside their mouths. When the cells of these lesions are analyzed with laboratory diagnostics, they are found to be rich in a specific type of blood cell called an *eosinophil.* The cause(s) of these lesions is unknown; however, they may be the result of a hypersensitivity or allergy. Some authorities feel they may arise as a result of an abnormality in the cat's own immune system. These are termed immune mediated disorders. It is very likely that the cause is a combination of an immune mediated disorder and a hypersensitivity reaction. Various names have been given to these bright red raw lesions. *Granulomas* about the *lips* are commonly referred to as *rodent ulcers* or simply lip ulcers (see figure 11-5). Well circumscribed lesions on the *inguinal* and *abdominal areas* are called *eosinophilic plaque* or *lick granulomas.* A *linear granuloma* is one type of lesion that may develop on the limbs, usually the rear. Another form of linear granuloma can develop inside the mouth on the tongue, gums and palate. Regardless of their names, eosinophilic ulcer, eosinophilic plaque and linear granulomas are all similar. Any age of cat may be affected. Because of their similarities, the treatments are often the same.

What Are the Symptoms?
The only symptom is the presence of a reddened inflamed-appearing lesion. The area will be devoid of hair. In most cases, the lesion(s) will be well defined. The lesion may be raised, "plaque-like" or eroded, forming an ulcer. Lesions may also develop inside the mouth.

What Are the Risks?
Usually these conditions are not life threatening and in many cases not even irritating to the patient, although in severe cases, ulcers in the mouth may hinder eating. If a cat has large or multiple lesions, it is possible for a bacterial infection to develop within the ulcerated tissue. This is not, however, a common occurrence.

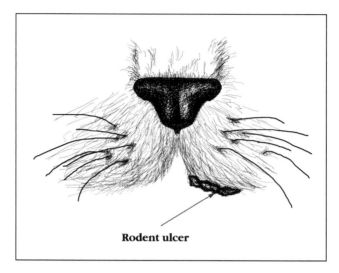

Rodent ulcer

11-5   Rodent ulcer

What Is the Treatment?

Many cats respond to various medications regardless of the exact type of granuloma. Steroids such as hydrocortisones are usually the drugs of choice. Methylprednisolone acetate (Depo-Medrol™) is usually administered by injection with good results expected. Progesterone compounds such as megestrol acetate (Ovaban) and Depo-Provera™ have provided a good response in some patients.

ABSCESSES

Abscesses under the skin are one of the most common ailments seen in cats. An abscess (sometimes referred to as a boil) is an area of infection, usually characterized by a painful, fluid-filled swelling. This is sometimes referred to as a pus. Any material that irritates the skin may cause an abscess to develop. Bite and scratch wounds from other cats are a cause, but thorns, hay, sticks, bee stings, flea bites and other biting insects can all break the skin, allowing bacteria to enter, resulting in an abscess formation.

What Are the Symptoms?

Usually the abscessed area will be swollen, reddened and painful to the touch. A visible wound may or may not be present. Most abscesses seen in cats tend to be about the head, neck and legs. This may be due to animals inflicting wounds on each other or to the fact that the head, neck and limbs are frequently exposed to the elements. Ninety percent of the time, the cause will not be determined.

What Are the Risks?

An abscess is an area of infection and, left untreated, the infection can spread to other areas of the body. The infectious bacteria can leave the abscess area and enter the bloodstream (septicemia), in which case death could result. This is seldom the case, however, and most abscesses remain localized.

What Is the Treatment?

The abscess, being fluid-filled, will occasionally rupture and drain. Once drained, they usually heal rapidly. If the abscess is large and not draining, veterinary intervention may be required. The abscess should be lanced and drained, and oral antibiotics may be required to fight infection. However, antibiotics will seldom work without sufficient drainage.

FROSTBITE

Frostbite is a term used to describe the damage to tissues due to an exposure to severely cold temperatures. Most healthy cats can easily withstand sub-zero temperatures provided they have shelter to remain dry and out of the wind. At the authors' hospital, most cats with frostbite are the result of other injuries, such as being struck by a car or caught in a fence. If a cat becomes disabled, it is exposed without protection to severe temperatures.

The body areas most likely to be frozen are the ears, tail and feet. Ninety percent of all cases treated by the authors had injury to the ears only, usually the tips or outer half of the ear flap.

What Are the Symptoms?

Initially, areas damaged from frostbite appear normal. Within 48 hours the damaged tissue will swell and become painful. Within seven days, due to the interruption of blood flow and nerve supply, the affected tissue dries up and turns black, eventually falling off.

What Are the Risks?

Frostbite may be minor or severe. Minor cases involve only the ear tips, whereas more extensive freezing causes the loss of the tail and appendages. Death may result if the limbs are involved. Dying tissue attracts bacteria, and severe, life-threatening infections can result.

What Is the Treatment?

If frostbite is suspected it is best to immediately warm the patient. Let the cat warm slowly at room or slightly-above-room temperature. Do not place the patient in hot water or in other areas of extreme temperatures. A gentle massaging of the affected areas may help increase blood flow and stimulate warming. Once warmed, consult a veterinarian. The amount of tissue damage will need to be assessed over a several day period. Dead tissue must be removed. The patient is usually placed on oral antibiotics to prevent infections.

INGROWN NAILS

Ingrown nails occur when the nail grows in a complete circle and penetrates back into the pad (see figure 11-6). It is more common in polydactyl cats. Polydactyl cats commonly have extra toes located on the side of the leg near the dew claw. These nails wear unevenly due to a lack of contact with the ground or floor.

What Are the Symptoms?
As they advance, ingrown nails will actually penetrate the skin and cause pain. The affected pet may limp or excessively lick the area in an attempt to alleviate the pain.

What Are the Risks?
The greatest risk associated with ingrown nails is the possible development of a secondary bacterial or fungal infection in the damaged skin.

What Is the Treatment?
Simple regular trimming of the nails is all that is required to prevent ingrown nails. Once ingrown, the nail(s) will need to be cut and sometimes surgically removed. Antibiotics will help eliminate a bacterial infection if present.

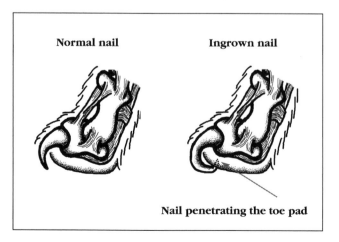

Normal nail   **Ingrown nail**

Nail penetrating the toe pad

11-6   Normal and ingrown nail

Disorders of the Ear

The feline ear serves a dual purpose. Its obvious function is, of course, hearing. But it is also extremely important as an organ of balance.

The **ear flap,** or pinna, is the portion of the ear that is most visible (see figure 12-1). Most cat's ears are erect; however, the Scottish Fold breeds have ear flaps that fold downward upon themselves. The ear flap serves as a partial covering of the ear canal, while at the same time directing sound towards the eardrum. The flap has an inner core of cartilage to give it strength. Both outer and inner surfaces of the skin are covered by hair, although hair follicles are much less prevalent on the inner areas.

The **ear canal** is a long tube-like structure that travels diagonally down the side of the head, then moves horizontally into the head. The total length of the canal is at least two inches, even in small breeds. The canal is circular and slightly smaller in diameter than a pencil. The length and size of the canal varies somewhat as to the feline's overall body size. As the ear canal passes into the head, it ends at a thin tissue called the tympanic membrane, or eardrum. This outer ear in the cat includes all structures, such as the canal and ear flap, from the eardrum outward. Internally, beyond the eardrum comes the middle ear (see figure 12-2), which is connected to the throat area by the eustachian tube. This tube allows air to enter the middle ear to balance the pressure against the eardrum.

Farther in from the **middle ear** is the **inner ear.** The inner ear maintains the cat's equilibrium, or balance. This structure contains fluid-filled canals, which tell the brain the exact body position as the fluid shifts. If a cat's head is tilted, the fluid shifts and the brain detects the tilting.

The hearing process starts when the eardrum picks up sound waves through air vibration. The **eardrum** vibrates and stimulates the bones in the middle ear. The vibrating bones pass the sound vibrations to an

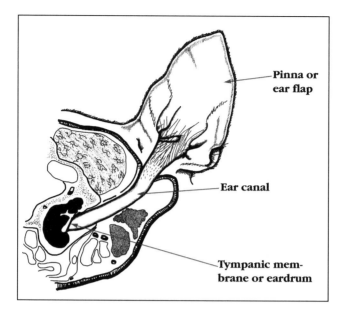

12-1 Ear

area containing tiny hairs. As the hairs move, sound waves are transformed to electrical impulses and then passed to the inner ear, where they are transmitted by the auditory nerve to the brain, where it is detected as sound.

The ear flap, canal, eardrum, and middle and inner ear all play important roles. These structures are complex and occasionally become diseased, thus impairing their function. Disorders of the ear are frequently very painful and can affect both hearing and equilibrium.

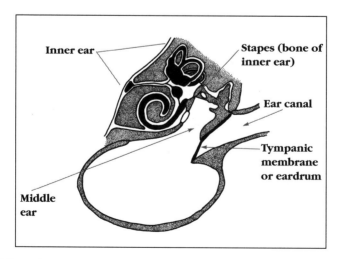

12-2 Middle and inner ear

AURICULAR HEMATOMA

As previously stated, the ear flap (pinna) is made up of two layers of skin with an inner core of cartilage. Numerous blood vessels and nerves extend from the inner vascular areas of the head all the way to the end of the pinna. Trauma to the ear flap can rupture or damage these delicate blood vessels. Trauma may be the result of a blow to the ear or a bite from another animal. Additionally, outer ear infections are very painful and may cause cats to violently scratch their ears. This scratching can also damage the ear flap.

If a major vessel within the ear flap ruptures, large amounts of blood can leak into the space between the skin and cartilage. This pool of blood is called a *hematoma*. The flap becomes very thick and may appear swollen, as the skin and cartilage are spread apart because of the hemorrhage (see figure 12-3).

What Are the Symptoms?
The most noted symptom is a large, fluid-filled cyst within the ear flap or pinna. Generally, cats will scratch about the ear. If an ear infection is also present, there may be an unpleasant odor coming from the ear canal as well.

What Are the Risks?
An auricular hematoma is not life threatening. Hematomas caused by ear infections are more serious than those caused by trauma because the underlying infection can cause hearing loss and severe discomfort. Untreated, these hematomas can become excessive in size, resulting in permanent damage to the pinna. If the cat severely scratches, the skin over the hematoma may tear, releasing the blood. This may stimulate further bleeding and increase the risk of infections.

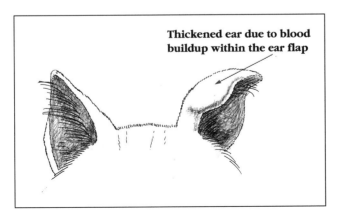

Thickened ear due to blood buildup within the ear flap

12-3   Auricular hematoma

What Is the Treatment?

Each patient with an auricular hematoma should have a careful examination to determine the cause. Was it caused by trauma from another cat, or was it the result of an ear infection? The underlying cause can then be treated. The blood-filled flap is usually surgically excised to remove the blood. Sutures are placed through the ear to hold the inner skin, cartilage and outer skin tightly together so that the space cannot refill with blood and the structures can heal back together. It must be emphasized that all auricular hematoma patients should be examined for deeper ear infections. In the authors' experience, 90 percent of all cases are caused by self trauma resulting from an ear infection.

INFECTIONS OF THE OUTER EAR (OTITIS EXTERNA)

Otitis externa describes an infection of the ear structures outside of the eardrum. The ear canal that extends from the ear flap to the eardrum is the structure diseased in otitis externa (see figure 12-4). Many organisms, including bacteria, yeasts and fungi, can affect the ear canals of the cat. Of the three, the most common pathogens are bacteria.

What Are the Symptoms?

Otitis externa can be present with a variety of symptoms and degrees. Generally, the most noted sign is head shaking and/or scratching at the head with a foot. Sometimes an odor will be detected. This is from the infection causing an excess of waxy secretions, and from the infection

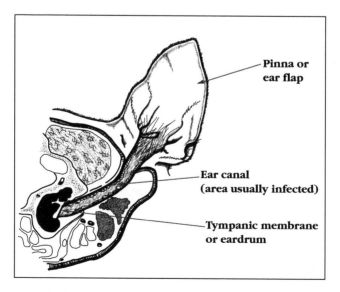

Pinna or ear flap

Ear canal (area usually infected)

Tympanic membrane or eardrum

12-4   Outer ear infections

itself. If cats are in extreme pain, they may refuse to eat. In severe infections, the canal will be damaged and bloody. Mild otitis externa may go undetected by the owner, only to be discovered upon a routine veterinary examination of the ear. In advanced cases, the ear canal becomes clogged with wax and fluid oozing from the tissues, and hearing may be impaired.

What Are the Risks?

All cases of otitis externa are potentially serious. Damage may extend to the eardrum, causing permanent hearing loss. If the drum is damaged, the infection may spread to the middle and inner ear, causing severe and permanent damage. Additionally, many animals will severely mutilate their ears when scratching themselves.

What Is the Treatment?

Otitis externa must be evaluated carefully to determine the cause. Veterinary diagnostic tests such as bacterial and fungal cultures can be performed.

Many ear ointments are available to kill bacteria, yeast and fungi. In very severe and chronic cases, surgery can be performed to "open up" and shorten the ear canal, thereby providing better drainage and drying of the sensitive tissues.

Many commercial solutions are available for routine use to help prevent infections. These washes or cleansing agents clean and dissolve ear wax and debris and dry the canals. Additionally, these slightly acidic solutions discourage the reproduction of bacteria, yeasts and fungal organisms. Good quality cleansing solutions, despite being acidic, are virtually sting-free. Affected pets should have their ears cleaned at least weekly with these solutions so that future infections can be avoided. A careful examination of the ear should be performed to identify the cause.

PARASITES OF THE OUTER EAR (EAR MITES)

Just as infectious organisms such as bacteria, yeast and fungi can invade the ear canal, so can parasites such as ear mites (see figure 12-5).

A little-known fact about ear mite infestations is that there are several types of mites that may invade the ears of cats. The most common is *Otodectes cynotis,* which probably accounts for 90 percent of the ear mite infestations. Other mites found in the ear canals of cats include *Notoedres cati, Demodex felis, Trombicula alfreddugesi* and the common mange mite *Sarcoptes scabiei.* All are mites and generally referred to simply as ear mites. Contrary to popular belief, ear mites do not live only in the ear. Mites move over the cat's entire body, migrating into the ear to feed.

What Are the Symptoms?

Cats with ear mites will scratch about the ears and/or shake their heads. The amount of scratching and shaking depends on the severity of the mite infestation. With more advanced infestations, the ear canals will bleed and either fresh or dried blood will appear inside the canal. Dried blood resembles coffee grounds. If you peer into your cat's ears and notice a buildup of "coffee grounds" material, then your cat probably has ear mites.

What Are the Risks?

Ear mites are very common, but still serious. Left untreated, they severely damage the ear canals and eardrum and can cause permanent hearing loss. Additionally, the mites are easily spread to other pets within the household including cats, dogs, rabbits, hamsters, gerbils, mice, ferrets, etc.

What Is the Treatment?

Various commercial ear preparations are available to kill the mites. These products contain an insecticide, usually pyrethrins. Ear products without an insecticide will not kill the mites. The ears may need to be

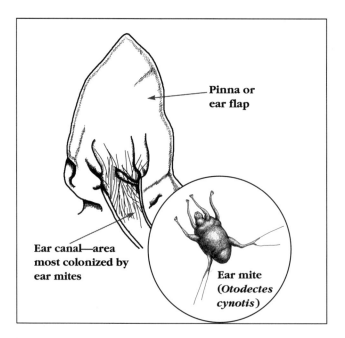

Pinna or ear flap

Ear canal—area most colonized by ear mites

Ear mite (*Otodectes cynotis*)

12-5   Ear mite

treated two to four weeks until all mites are killed. As previously mentioned, many ear mites live all over the body, including the feet and tail. These areas should also be treated. Most products designed for fleas and ticks, including sprays, dips and shampoos, will be effective. Be sure to treat the tail. This is because while sleeping, the tail is curled around the cat's body and frequently lies in close contact with the ear. Because mites are very easily transferred between pets, it is best if all pets in the household receive simultaneous treatment. Most types of mites do not survive long off the pets, so the treatment of the house and yard usually is not necessary.

INFECTIONS OF THE MIDDLE EAR (OTITIS MEDIA)

Otitis media describes an infection of the middle ear or the area immediately inside the eardrum (see figure 12-6). Generally, otitis media develops as a result of infections in the ear canal. The eardrum becomes damaged and bacteria (rarely funguses) enter the middle ear through the damaged eardrum. This infection can also rise from bacteria carried there by the bloodstream or when they make their way up the throat via the eustachian tube.

What Are the Symptoms?

Head shaking, scratching at the head and ear area and difficulty hearing are indications of a middle ear infection. Since major nerves supplying the facial muscles pass through the middle ear, the facial muscles

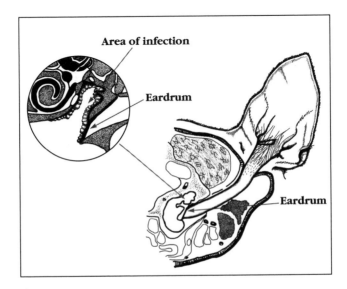

12-6 Middle ear infection

can also be affected. Since the jaw bones of the cat extend behind the ear, pain may be evident when the cat's mouth is opened. A foul-smelling discharge may be present in the ear canal if the eardrum has ruptured. In cases of middle ear infection where the eardrum remains intact, it will appear discolored and bulging outward on examination.

What Are the Risks?

Because the middle ear is closely associated with major nerves and is principally responsible for hearing, all infections are considered serious. There is also the chance of damage to the eardrum.

What Is the Treatment?

Most infections of the middle ear are bacterial in nature and respond to oral antibiotics. Flushing the ear canal to cleanse the outer and middle ear is beneficial. Due to pain, anesthesia is generally required to flush the middle ear. A culture done on the draining material will reveal the cause; although usually bacterial, fungi are occasionally diagnosed as the culprit. Cases not responsive to oral medications and flushing may require surgery to open and clean out the area. Medical therapy may need to be ongoing for several months until a cure can be achieved.

FOREIGN BODIES IN THE EAR CANAL

The ear canal drops downward before it enters into the head horizontally. It is therefore a convenient place to collect or catch foreign material such as weeds, sticks, seeds and dirt. The most frequent foreign bodies found in the ear are bits of weeds and grasses.

What Are the Symptoms?

Generally, the foreign materials irritate or tickle the ear canal. The patients usually shake their heads or scratch at their ears.

What Are the Risks?

Most foreign bodies simply irritate the canal. However, they can occasionally puncture the eardrum. They pose no real threat unless the eardrum is damaged. Once these objects are removed, the patient quickly recovers.

What Is the Treatment?

All foreign bodies should be removed at once. Often they are deep within the canal and can be seen only with a special ear scope (otoscope). Removal may require specialized instruments capable of reaching deep into the canal, which in some cases may require anesthesia.

HEREDITARY DEAFNESS

Hereditary deafness, occasionally referred to as neonatal deafness, begins at birth. A cat with hereditary deafness will be born with normal ears, but within a few days of birth, structures important for hearing within the ear degenerate. When the kitten's ear canals open up a few weeks later, the kitten is deaf.

The gene for deafness is the same gene required for a white coat color; however, deafness is not evident in every white kitten. In reality, most white kittens are not deaf, but most deaf kittens are white. *It appears that long-haired white cats are more likely to be deaf than white cats with short hair.*

White cats may have yellow or blue eyes, and occasionally one eye of each color. A cat with one eye of each color is often referred to as an odd-eyed cat. While cats with any of the above three eye combinations may be deaf, most commonly, it is those with blue eyes or one blue eye that are affected.

Although we refer to this condition as a deafness, many of these cats are not completely deaf. Occasionally only one ear is affected while the other ear remains normal. An odd-eyed white cat (one blue eye and one yellow) very commonly is deaf only in the blue-eyed side with normal hearing on the yellow-eyed side.

Cats with hereditary deafness should not be bred. Breeding deaf white cats greatly increases the odds of the kittens being deaf.

Again, it should be understood that most white cats, even those with blue eyes, are not deaf. Many have normal hearing, or at least normal hearing in one ear, so they are only partially deaf. Simply put, white cats with blue eyes have a greater than normal chance of deafness when compared to other colored cats, but most white cats with blue eyes have normal hearing.

DEAFNESS AND AGING

Deafness associated with aging is common in the feline. As the patient ages, the eardrum and nerves associated with hearing deteriorate, leading to some degree of hearing deficit. Fortunately, the hearing loss progresses gradually and seldom seriously affects the pet's well-being. There is no way to predict the full extent or rapidity of the deafness. No medications are available to reverse the progression of symptoms.

Deafness associated with aging is simply part of the normal aging process and is seen in at least 50 percent of all geriatric patients.

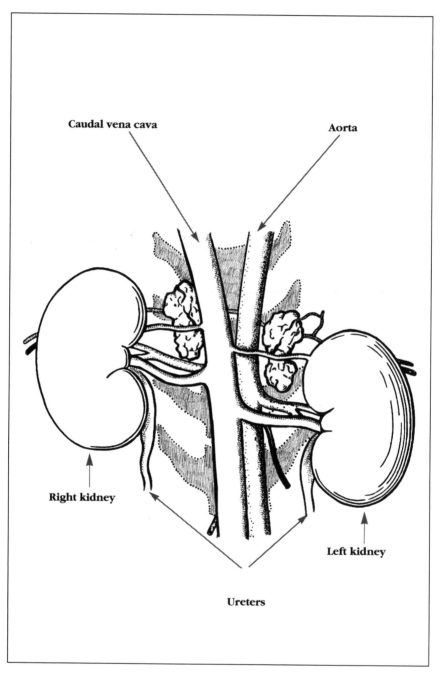

Caudal vena cava

Aorta

Right kidney

Left kidney

Ureters

13-1　Kidneys

CHAPTER 13

The Urinary System

Metabolism is the process of cells *burning* nutrients for fuel, while at the same time *building* larger particles, such as proteins from amino acids. Additionally, as the body works, cells die and release their contents into the body on a daily basis. Both metabolism and cellular death create waste materials such as excess nitrogen and phosphorus that would poison the body if they were not eliminated.

The urinary system detects, filters and removes toxic wastes in the blood, and finally excretes them from the body.

The two **kidneys** filter wastes from the blood and combine it with water to form urine (see figure 13-1). The urine passes from the kidneys down small muscular tubes called **ureters,** which empty into the **bladder.** The bladder is a balloon-like structure bound with muscle. It functions as a storage site for urine until it can be eliminated from the body. When the bladder empties, urine flows down the **urethra** and out the body. The male and female urinary systems are very similar. The closely associated organs of reproduction that differ are covered in Chapter 1, "The Feline Reproductive System."

DISORDERS OF THE KIDNEYS AND URETERS

The kidneys are large, bean-shaped organs; one is on the right side of the body and the other is on the left. Both are just under the backbone immediately behind the rib cage. Every drop of blood circulating through the vessels of the body passes, through the kidneys. Kidneys are composed of a complex network of minute blood vessels and specialized blood "filters" called *glomeruli*. The kidneys don't really filter blood, but rather they select certain nutrients to remain within the blood while extracting others in the formation of urine. Calcium and sodium are two examples of substances the kidneys conserve and keep within the blood. On the other hand, very little nitrogen and phosphorus are saved, hence most is passed out with the urine. Because of its high nitrogen content, a cat's urine burns the grass and creates yellow spots on the lawn. Kidneys also detect the proper amount of water to leave in the blood. Excess fluid is removed from the bloodstream by the kidneys and becomes a component of urine. If a pet drinks excess amounts then the kidneys will produce more than normal amounts of urine.

Nitrogen is a primary component of urine. When a pet eats, the body converts protein and other substances into sugar to be used as fuel. Proteins contain nitrogen while sugar does not. Nitrogen then becomes a waste product of protein digestion; by itself nitrogen is toxic to cells. Excess nitrogen, is continually removed from the blood by the kidneys and excreted into the urine. Blood tests performed by veterinarians frequently monitor the **b**lood **u**rea **n**itrogen levels (BUN) to indicate kidney function. Diseased kidneys cannot remove the excess nitrogen, so it reaches elevated proportions in the bloodstream. Higher than normal nitrogen levels in the bloodstream are not a result of eating too much protein, but rather the kidney's inability to excrete the nitrogen.

Because patients with diseased kidneys have a decreased ability to excrete nitrogen, low-protein diets are recommended for these patients. The lower the quantity of protein fed, the less nitrogen waste is produced. It is often erroneously believed that high-protein diets can damage the kidneys. This is not the case. Normal functioning kidneys can easily remove nitrogen produced from high-protein foods. In fact, patients with only one kidney can accomplish this task. High-protein foods are not the cause of kidney disease in the feline.

One generally unknown function of the kidneys is hormone production; a very important hormone called erythropoietin stimulates red blood cell production by the bone marrow. Failing kidneys may produce inadequate quantities of erythropoietin hormone, resulting in abnormally low levels of red cells in the blood (anemia).

ACUTE RENAL DISEASE

Acute renal disease is a kidney disorder that occurs suddenly. Possible causes include bacterial infections, drug toxicities from such substances as Gentamicin (an antibiotic), or poisons that contain ethylene glycol such as antifreeze. Despite the cause, the kidneys rapidly lose their ability to function correctly.

What Are the Symptoms?

Many symptoms of renal disease are caused by toxic nitrogen levels within the bloodstream. This is referred to as azotemia or uremia. Signs of azotemia include mouth ulcers, vomiting, seizures, diarrhea, bleeding disorders and depression. Diseased kidneys not only cannot excrete excess nitrogen, they also cannot conserve normal amounts of water. Body fluids are lost to the urine, resulting in dehydration. Signs of dehydration include dry or sticky gums and loss of skin elasticity. If one picks up the skin behind the neck of a normal patient, it will quickly snap back to normal; in the dehydrated patient the skin will remain elevated and "tent-like."

What Are the Risks?

Any disorder of the kidneys should be considered serious. Since most cases of acute renal disease have known causes, treatment can usually be successful.

What Is the Treatment?

Proper treatment is decided once the cause is identified. Intravenous fluids may be necessary to flush out the kidneys and supply needed fluids for the body. Any kidney-harming drugs should be discontinued. If a bacteria is suspected, then the appropriate antibiotic will usually eliminate the infection. It is very important to begin treatment early to prevent permanent damage from occurring to the delicate kidney tissues.

CHRONIC RENAL DISEASE

Chronic renal disease often has no identifiable cause. It is generally related to aging and is simply a deterioration and loss of filtration within the kidney. These "filters" are called glomeruli. When a significant portion of the glomeruli die or are injured, there may not be enough to remove normal wastes from the bloodstream and toxic levels of these substances develop within the body. Additionally, the kidneys can no longer conserve water. Abnormally large amounts of urine are produced, and needed water is lost from the body.

What Are the Symptoms?

Unlike acute renal disease, the signs of chronic renal disease develop slowly over time. Due to the inability of the kidneys to conserve water, one will frequently notice an increased urination both in frequency and volume. In an attempt to keep the body hydrated, the patient will compensate by consuming larger quantities of water. In the early stages of the disease, the nitrogen levels may or may not be elevated in the bloodstream. The kidneys can lose more than 75 percent of their normal function before they are no longer capable of detoxifying the body. If the nitrogen is elevated in the blood (azotemia), then mouth ulcers may develop in addition to weight loss, poor appetite, bleeding disorders and possible seizures. The early warning signs are an increased thirst and urination followed by symptoms of azotemia. In severe cases, due to a lack of the hormone erythropoietin, there may be a decreased production of red blood cells and anemia.

What Are the Risks?

Many older patients have some degree of kidney failure. Mildly affected patients will live relatively normal lives. They compensate for their loss of kidney function by drinking excess quantities of water to flush their system. More severely affected patients will not be able to cope with the loss of kidney function and may die from renal failure. Renal failure is number one of the "natural causes" of death in the feline. Unlike humans, the feline heart generally out-performs the kidneys of the individual animal.

What Is the Treatment?

Most cases of chronic renal disease and failure are not reversible. The kidneys have simply worn out. If the early signs of diseased kidneys are recognized before they actually fail (i.e., increased thirst and urination), there are treatments to help slow down this degenerative process of the kidneys. The feeding of low-protein diets will reduce the dietary intake of nitrogen and therefore decrease the workload of the kidneys. Commercially prepared diets are available from veterinarians. Again, diets high in protein do not initially cause kidney problems or disease. This is often inferred because low-protein diets are used in the management of renal disease.

INHERITED POLYCYSTIC KIDNEYS

Kidney disease is a disorder usually associated with middle-aged and older cats; however, inherited polycystic kidneys affect young cats and kittens. Although not common, this disorder is included here as it can be hereditary and surface within familial lines. One or both kidneys may be involved. With inherited polycystic kidney disease, large fluid-filled cysts form in the kidney and crowd out the normal kidney tissue. This leads to a death of the normal kidney cells and loss of kidney function.

What Are the Symptoms?

The symptoms are the same as those associated with chronic renal disease; however, the age of onset is younger. The symptoms associated with inherited polycystic kidneys will generally occur in patients under two years of age and may be as young as eight weeks. Upon examination, the kidney(s) initially appear greatly enlarged due to the cysts. As the kidneys scar and begin to fail, they may shrink to a smaller-than-normal size.

What Are the Risks?

Most patients with polycystic kidney disease will live a shortened life span. Many die before reaching maturity. The seriousness depends on whether one or both kidneys are abnormal, and to what extent they are diseased.

What Is the Treatment?

There is no totally corrective treatment for inherited polycystic kidney disease. In rare instances, surgery is performed to remove the cysts and spare the normal kidney tissue. *Even with surgical treatment, the long-term prognosis is poor.*

KIDNEY CANCER

As with many organs within the body, tumors may invade the kidney(s). Several types of tumors have been isolated from the kidneys of cats. Tumors may develop only in the kidneys, or they may be the result of a spread of cancer from elsewhere within the body.

What Are the Symptoms?

The symptoms are very similar to those associated with a chronic renal disease. Upon examination by a trained hand, the tumors or "lumps" may be felt on the kidney's surface.

What Are the Risks?

Cancer of the kidney(s) is always serious. Often, upon further exploration tumors are found in other areas of the body as well. Usually a complete cure is not possible.

What Is the Treatment?

Surgery is the of choice for kidney cancer. If only one kidney is involved, it can be totally removed (nephrectomy) to eliminate the tumor and diseased kidney. Many patients can live fairly normal lives with only one functioning kidney. Although surgery helps in a few cases, many times cancer is simultaneously found elsewhere, either in the other kidney or other organs. In instances where both kidneys and/or other organs are involved, the prognosis may be very poor. The exact type of cancer should be determined with a biopsy to help define the expected outcome and long-term prognosis.

DISORDERS OF THE BLADDER AND URETHRA

The bladder is a balloon-like structure surrounded by layers of muscle. Its primary function is the storage of urine. Each kidney has one **ureter,** which deposits urine into the bladder. From the bladder, urine exits the body through the **urethra.** The **urethral opening** is at the end of the male *penis* and within the *vagina* of the female (see figure 13-2). Contrary to popular belief, urine is neither dirty nor contaminated. In fact, normal urine is sterile until it exits the body. The bladder, even though it is basically a storage unit for sterile urine, does commonly become diseased.

CYSTITIS—INFECTION OF THE BLADDER

Cystitis describes a situation in which the bladder has become inflamed. Commonly this is due to bacteria that have entered the bladder from the outside, usually through the urethra, thereby resulting in an infection. Female cats have a shorter and wider urethra than males and this probably contributes to the fact that most bladder infections are found in females. Bacteria have an easier access to the female bladder.

What Are the Symptoms?
Frequent urination is the most common sign associated with an infection of the bladder. The bladder becomes painful when irritated, and therefore the patient urinates more in an attempt to keep the bladder empty. The act of urination may be painful, and cause a burning sensation. The patient starts to urinate but quits, only to try again within a short time. Occasionally urine accidents may happen in unwanted areas, such as around the house. If the cause is a severe bacterial infection, then blood may appear in the urine.

What Are the Risks?
Normally, the urine and the organ it passes through are sterile, or free from bacteria. If bacteria have entered the bladder, it is possible for infections to not only affect that area, but the kidneys as well. Kidney

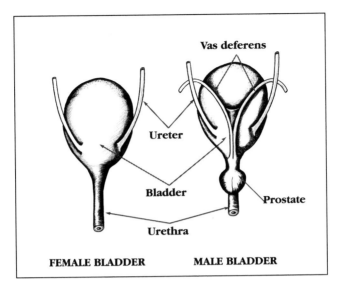

13-2   Female and male bladder

infections are rare, but very serious. Suspected cases of cystitis should be treated at once.

What Is the Treatment?

Bladder infections are generally caused by bacteria. A culture of the urine will reveal the bacteria type. Excellent antibiotics are now available to treat many bacterial infections that affect the bladder. Occasionally, drugs are given in addition to antibiotics to help lower the pH (increasing the acidity) of the urine. This is done because bacteria do not thrive in acidic urine.

URETHRITIS

Urethritis is simply an irritation of the urethra. As in humans, many of these are bacterial in origin. Infection of the urethra often accompanies bladder infection (cystitis).

What Are the Symptoms?

The act of urination may create a burning sensation and cause the patient to stop urinating once it begins. A thick yellow discharge may be noted at the urethral opening.

What Are the Risks?

Urethral infections are seldom serious. They should, however, be promptly treated to prevent the bacteria from entering the bladder and causing an infection there.

What Is the Treatment?

Infections of the urethra generally respond well to antibiotics. A culture of the urine and/or urethral discharge will reveal the bacterial type. This is especially important in breeding animals to decrease the likelihood of transmitting the infection sexually.

URINARY CALICULI (URINARY STONES OR UROLITHIASIS)

In the feline, small "sand-like" crystals can occasionally form within the urine. The crystals may clump together and form caliculi or stones. In contrast to humans, this rarely occurs in the kidneys of the feline. In cats, crystal and stone formations principally occur within the bladder. The crystals may be small, and similar to sand, or they may clump into larger aggregates called stones and be as large as several inches in diameter (see figure 13-3).

The cause of urinary caliculi formation is unknown. Some patients simply seem more prone to it. There are many dissolved salts in the urine of a cat. When these salts combine, stones are formed. It is generally believed that it's not the excess salts in the diet that are the cause of stone formation, but rather it's the way the body metabolizes salts and other products.

Complex laboratory analysis of urinary stones has isolated several different types in the feline, including struvite, oxalate and ammonium urate. Struvite caliculi, which is a mixture of magnesium and ammonium phosphate, is the most common. It should be noted that some

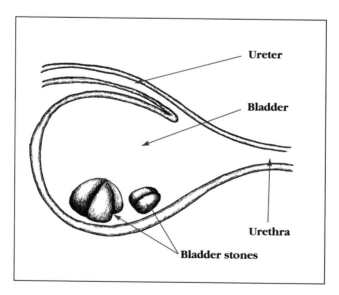

13-3   Bladder stones

authorities refer to struvite crystals as phosphates. All are stones comprised of various elements and may include magnesium, calcium, phosphate and ammonia. Some types of stones form more quickly in acid urines (pH less than 7.0) while others prefer more alkaline urines (higher pH). Acidic urine discourages the formation of struvite and ammonium urate crystals, but favors calcium oxalate crystal formation. Although urine acidity can help predict the stone type, only a laboratory analysis of the stone can conclusively identify its type.

What Are the Symptoms?

Despite their differences in composition, urinary caliculi present similar signs. Stones in the bladder will irritate the bladder's inner lining and cause painful urination. Additionally, the bladder wall may bleed and produce noticeable amounts of blood in the urine. Stones, particularly large ones, occupy a significant space within the bladder. This limits the amount of urine the bladder can retain. Due to this, the patient may urinate small quantities with increased frequency. Bladder infections, or cystitis, may develop as a result of bladder and urethra damage caused by the crystals and/or stones. The common signs are: frequent urination that is often painful, blood within the urine, urine leakage, and a painful abdomen.

What Are the Risks?

Urinary stones are always serious. The worst instance involves cases where small stones become lodged within the urethra and obstruct normal urination. A patient with an inability to urinate will usually die within 48 hours. *Difficulty urinating is always an emergency.*

What Is the Treatment?

Treatment varies with each individual. Surgery is often necessary to remove stones formed within the bladder and/or urethra. In some cases, special commercially prepared diets can be used that dissolve the stones while they are in the bladder. During or after removal, medications may help alter the urine pH. Some products lower the pH, making the urine more acidic. This will discourage the formation of stones such as struvite and urate crystals. Other medications raise the urine pH, making the urine more alkaline. This discourages stones such as calcium oxalate from developing. Diets low in elements such as magnesium have been used to help reduce struvite crystal formation. A careful analysis of each patient and stone type is necessary to determine the proper treatment.

FELINE UROLOGICAL SYNDROME (FUS)

Feline urological syndrome, simply referred to as FUS, is the most common urinary tract ailment of felines. In fact, it is the most common medical reason that a cat sees the veterinarian. Both males and females, spayed and unspayed, are affected. As many as one in twenty adult cats will develop this disease during their lifetime. The syndrome itself is generally not severe, but it is serious and life-threatening consequences can develop. A thorough understanding of the disorder is necessary so that early warning signs can be detected. Treatment and prevention should be initiated at once.

FUS is often misunderstood. It is not just a disease of neutered cats; it is very common in unneutered males and even females as well. Likewise, neutering male cats at a young age does not predispose them to develop FUS. The most serious consequences will, however, usually involve male cats. The reason for this will be explained in more detail later.

There is no single known cause for FUS and many factors seem to be involved. These may include genetics, diet, exercise, season of the year, bacteria, and possibly even a virus component. It is best described as a disorder of the bladder that includes urinary crystal formation; blood in the urine; bladder inflammation; frequent, difficult urination; an occasional inability to urinate; and possibly an infection. Crystal formation in the urine is the most serious development and probably results in the other signs mentioned above.

A cat with FUS will have small, sugar-like crystals that form within the urine. These crystals are made up of several minerals including magnesium and calcium. The reason why these crystals develop is unclear, but it may be linked to the individual cat's ability (or lack of ability) to use magnesium from ingested foods. Viruses of the bladder have long been suspected of causing crystal formation, but this has never been proven. Genetics may play a role in regulating how an individual cat metabolizes and excretes magnesium; we have not, however, noticed a familial or breed tendency toward crystal formation.

When crystals form in the bladder, its walls and urethral surfaces become irritated and inflamed. The urine will usually be visibly blood-stained. The crystals can form stones that range up to the size of a marble. Smaller stones will readily pass from the bladder into the urethra. That is the source of a life-threatening situation.

The urethra is a small, narrow tube through which urine is discharged from the bladder. In the female it remains large from the time it leaves the bladder until it exits the body. In the male, the urethra narrows as it enters the penis. It is within the penis that small stones finally lodge, and cause a complete or partial obstruction that prevents the cat from being able to urinate. This blocked or plugged cat will die within 48 hours if left untreated.

It is a false belief that the urethra of a neutered cat is narrower than that of an unneutered tom. In fact, some neutered males have a larger, more "female-like" urethra. It is true that most cases of blocked cats occur in neutered males, but that is simply because the majority of male pet cats are neutered. Females very rarely block because their larger urethra easily allows the crystals to pass. Still, they are also susceptible to FUS.

For unknown reasons, nearly 90 percent of all cats with FUS will develop signs of the disease in the spring. In our hospital, February and March have the highest occurrence. This may be linked to poor exercise habits during the winter months or a decrease in water consumption during cooler periods. An increase in water consumption in the heat of summer may result in a flushing or cleansing out of the bladder before crystals reach a size that can cause problems.

What Are the Symptoms?
The signs of a cat suffering with FUS are usually easily detected. The hallmark is "crying" while trying to urinate. Also if the cat associates the pain with the litter box, he or she may begin to urinate in other areas. Any cat that suddenly stops urinating in a litter box is cause for concern. Be sure to differentiate between this behavior and that of spraying, a habit of marking territory. Spraying takes place on vertical objects such as walls and curtains. Urination will take place on flat, horizontal surfaces such as the top of a bed, in the bathtub, on the carpet or rugs. In any event, any abnormal urinary habit can indicate FUS.

A cat suffering from FUS will cry from pain while attempting to urinate. Owners should not confuse this sign with constipation, which is rare in the cat. The abdomen of an FUS cat will become enlarged and often even an untrained hand can detect the hard, orange-sized mass of the distended bladder. In advanced stages, the cat will appear weak and delirious.

What Are the Risks?
As previously discussed, FUS in which the patient is unable to urinate is life threatening. Within 48 hours of blockage, the patient will die from kidney shutdown. Any cat with any degree of FUS should be monitored closely, as blockage could occur at any time.

What Is the Treatment?
Treatment and prevention of FUS is varied, but a few basic principles apply. First, the blocked cat is a medical emergency to be treated without delay. This patient will be catheterized to remove the blocking

stones, thus allowing a normal flow of urine. In severe or reoccurring cases, a surgery called perineal urethrostomy will be performed. This surgery removes the male organ and creates a larger, more female-like urethra. This patient may still develop FUS, but rarely will again become blocked.

Additionally, antibiotics are usually administered to a cat with FUS to kill or remove any bacteria within the bladder. It is not known whether bacteria are a direct cause of the disease or merely the result of damage to the organs by the crystals, but a patient with the disease will occasionally have a bacterial infection of the bladder called cystitis. It is known that most urinary crystals that cause FUS will form most easily in urine with a high pH (alkaline urine). Oral urinary acidifiers such as Methigel paste are commonly given to cats with a history of FUS. The principle here is that by maintaining an acidic urine, both crystal formation and bacterial growth will be inhibited.

Although the use of acidifiers is common, the benefit is scientifically unclear. Other research has gone into the formulation of low magnesium diets in an attempt to decrease the incidence of FUS. This is sometimes referred to as "ash content." After a food is burned, what remains is called "ash." Ash is a compound of many elements including calcium, phosphorous, magnesium and others. Magnesium is the key component of urinary crystals, and today's literature will usually refer to low magnesium diets rather than low ash diets.

Since other elements are present, it is possible to have high ash, yet low magnesium content. *Again, the magnesium, not the ash, is the culprit.* We know that a cat's tissues do not manufacture magnesium so the source must be dietary. It is well documented that low-magnesium diets will, to some extent, reduce the incidence of FUS, but it does not always eliminate or prevent it. The important point is that a low-magnesium diet is only part of a complicated puzzle.

Most commercially prepared cat foods are naturally low in magnesium, and supplements such as Torula yeast are lower in this ingredient than are the traditional feline supplements. Since cats seldom develop high blood pressure, salt is actually used as an aid to treat and prevent FUS. By lightly salting the daily meal, an increase in thirst occurs. A cat that consumes more water will produce more urine, which helps to continually flush the bladder and thus reduce crystal formation.

Whenever your cat uses areas other than the litter box, it is cause for concern. If it is FUS, the sooner treatment is initiated, the easier it is to cure. Additionally, if the problem continues for too long, behavior changes can occur that few owners can tolerate. Fortunately, despite lack of knowledge regarding the exact causes, we can still manage the condition and maintain quality health in cats with FUS.

C H A P T E R   1 4

The Lymphatic System

The lymphatic system filters and removes debris from the body. It is important in providing the body with immunity against diseases, as it can produce cells to fight infections.

The lymphatic system is composed of small circular *glands* called **lymph nodes** (see figure 14-1). The lymph nodes are connected to each other by a series of *vessels* called **lymphatics.** The lymphatics make up a large network of vessels throughout the body. The *liquid* they carry is referred to as **lymph.** The lymph nodes filter out cellular waste products and foreign material. Waste is then carried by the lymphatics to the chest of the animal where the material enters the bloodstream for excretion from the body.

The **lymph nodes** are glandular structures that produce disease-fighting white blood cells called *lymphocytes.* Lymphocytes circulate in the bloodstream to aid the immune response in various diseases. Other cells in the lymph nodes, called "B" cells, secrete small disease-fighting proteins called antibodies. Antibodies bind with foreign particles called *antigens* and help inactivate them. The **lymph glands** also act as filters to remove potentially dangerous infectious particles from the bloodstream. The **spleen** is the largest organ in the lymphatic system (see figure 14-2). It acts as a storage unit for red corpuscles and also as a blood filter. In summary, the lymphatic system is extremely important in providing the body immunity against diseases.

LYMPHOSARCOMA (LYMPHOMA)

Lymphosarcoma is a cancer of the lymph nodes. In cats, it is one of the most common cancers encountered. Viral diseases, most notably **feline leukemia virus** (FeLV), are known to trigger cancers of the lymph nodes in cats.

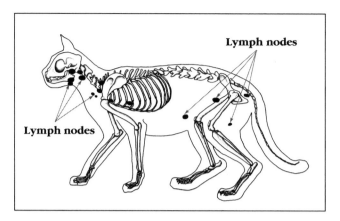

14-1 Lymph system

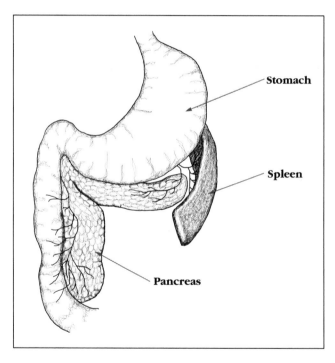

14-2 Spleen

What Are the Symptoms?

A cat with lymphosarcoma will experience severe weight loss. The lymph nodes may swell to the size of a marble or larger. Commonly, the bone marrow is also creating a lower-than-normal level of red and white blood cells. The gums and eyelids may appear pale rather than pink.

What Are the Risks?

Lymphosarcoma is serious and invariably fatal. An early diagnosis and treatment may slightly increase the life expectancy, but usually only by weeks to months. It is important in a cat with lymphosarcoma to search for the underlying cause. This will not only help select the treatment and prognosis, but help determine if the patient is contagious to other cats. Feline leukemia virus (FeLV) is extremely contagious by direct contact. Known cats carrying FeLV should be strictly isolated from healthy cats. For a more complete discussion of FeLV, refer to Chapter 16, "Infectious Feline Diseases."

What Is the Treatment?

Normally, a biopsy of one or more lymph nodes will confirm the diagnosis of lymphosarcoma. Various chemotherapeutic agents can be administered to fight the cancer. Anti-inflammatory medications such as prednisone are frequently used in conjunction with stronger chemotherapeutic agents. With treatment, some patients can survive a year or more.

At this point in veterinary medicine, we are rarely able to cure these patients. Therapy is aimed at upgrading the quality of life for several months to a year.

Common Feline Parasites

The term parasite is best described as an organism that draws its nourishment from another organism. In the cat, there are parasites that affect different areas of the body. **Ectoparasites** are found outside of the body and feed upon the skin. Classic examples of two feline ectoparasites are *fleas* and *ear mites*. **Endoparasites,** on the other hand, are those found within the body. Examples of endoparasites are *lungworms* that reside within the lungs and intestinal parasites such as *tapeworms, roundworms, coccidia* and *Toxoplasma.*

Parasites are always a cause for concern to the pet owner. In the cat, parasites can affect virtually every body system, and some parasites are carriers of other parasites. Fleas, for example, serve as a reservoir for some types of tapeworms.

Although some parasites are not overly serious from a medical standpoint, no cat is considered healthy if heavily infested with parasites. To maintain healthy cats, it is essential that the owner recognize at least some of the signs of the major parasites. For parasite treatment and prevention to be effective, a thorough knowledge of the parasitic life cycle and their vulnerability must be understood. It is also important to know which parasites are contagious to other household pets and to humans.

The authors have selected certain parasites for discussion in this book. These organisms were included either because they are common, pose serious health risks or are rarely understood and need clarification. Unfortunately, many parasites fit in all three categories.

PARASITES OF THE SKIN AND EARS

FLEAS

Fleas belong to the order Siphonaptera. Fleas are classified as insects because their bodies are divided into three parts: the head, thorax and abdomen. Attached to the thorax are three pairs of legs for a total of six. Fleas have no wings. The most noted flea characteristics are their medium brown color and laterally flattened body. They are slightly smaller than a sesame seed. The last pair of legs is sufficiently large to equip them with fantastic jumping ability. They feed on a wide range of hosts from many different kinds of warm-blooded animals.

Contrary to popular belief, every flea is not just a flea. In North America, there are at least seven different types. They prefer to live separately and do not interbreed. *Xenopsylla cheopis,* commonly known as the rat flea, is a carrier of bubonic plague. The name "rat flea" implies that rats are the preferred dinner, but cats will also do. *Nosopsyllus facets* also like rats, especially Norwegian and black rats. This flea is commonly called the European rat flea. The third type of flea is *Echidnophaga gallinacea,* also known as the tropical hen flea or the sticktight flea. It prefers to feast upon birds, but will also dine on cats. The squirrel flea bears the scientific name *Orchopeas howardii* and is generally found on squirrels, rodents and other animals, including cats.

Humans, despite self-proclaimed grace, have their own flea. Its scientific name is *Poleax aerations,* but it's referred to simply as the human flea. This flea also likes swine, as humans and swine biologically have much in common. However, if neither pigs nor people are available, it will feast on cats. Cats also have their own flea, named *Ctenocephalides felis.* This is the domestic cat flea, but it actually prefers dogs.

The larval stages of the dog and cat tapeworm, *Dipylidium caninum,* can reside within a flea's laterally flattened body. If your pet is harboring tapeworms, they were most likely contracted by the cat eating a flea that was carrying tapeworm. This flea will also bite humans. Its bites are small and painless, but do itch. Dogs have their own flea, classified as *Ctenocephalides canis,* but known simply as the common dog flea. Despite its name, it also feeds on humans, cats and other animals. It too carries tapeworms.

Problems in controlling flea numbers are due to their ability to live off of the hosts for long periods of time and their amazing reproductive abilities (see figure 15-1). In a normal situation they will take a blood meal and then immediately drop off the animal and reside in the carpet or grass. Fleas can also mate while off or on their host, and a single female will lay hundreds of eggs in a single day. These tiny, white eggs can be readily seen with only slight magnification. The female flea deposits these eggs both on and off the host, but those deposited on the host will drop to the carpet, bedding, grass or any areas underneath the pets.

Adult female—The female produces from 3 to 18 eggs at a time, laying them among her feces for the emerging larva to feed upon. With frequent feedings she may lay several hundred in her year life span.

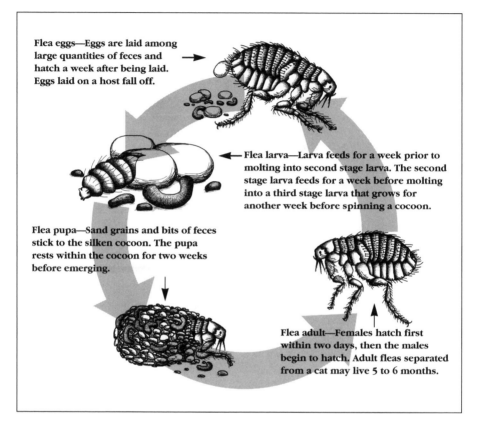

Flea eggs—Eggs are laid among large quantities of feces and hatch a week after being laid. Eggs laid on a host fall off.

Flea larva—Larva feeds for a week prior to molting into second stage larva. The second stage larva feeds for a week before molting into a third stage larva that grows for another week before spinning a cocoon.

Flea pupa—Sand grains and bits of feces stick to the silken cocoon. The pupa rests within the cocoon for two weeks before emerging.

Flea adult—Females hatch first within two days, then the males begin to hatch. Adult fleas separated from a cat may live 5 to 6 months.

15-1   Life cycle of a flea

It takes the spherical eggs about seven days to hatch into tiny infant fleas, called larvae. Larvae are not mobile enough to feed on pets; their diet consists entirely of flea feces from the adult. These feces are deposited into the carpeting, grass, bedding, etc. Depending on temperature and moisture, larvae exist for a variable length of time, but usually within two weeks of hatching they form a cocoon and enter the resting pupa stage. They remain in the cocoon for up to two weeks, upon which time they emerge as an adult. From egg to adult averages about 21 days, thus completing an entire generation. Fleas have the ability to explode in numbers under favorable conditions. Adult fleas feed upon the blood of their victims, but an adult flea can survive one full year without eating. Please remember this fact, as it is important in flea control.

What Are the Symptoms?

The most common symptom of a flea infestation is seeing the actual fleas or feces of the fleas. Flea feces resemble pepper upon the hair coat and are composed of digested blood. When placed in water the flea feces emit a red pigment. This helps in differentiating flea feces (flea dirt) from other types of debris, such as sand. Hair loss and itching may be evident on the flea-infested patient. Most animals itch and scratch around the back and rump. Occasionally, a patient has a severe allergic reaction to the flea saliva and may intensely itch after the bite of a single flea. This allergic reaction can be triggered by as little as three flea bites per month. It is important to know that *your pet does not need a lot of fleas to be miserable.*

What Are the Risks?

In the non-allergic cat, fleas do not always pose a serious health risk in terms of creating itching or creating an allergic response. Fleas are bloodsuckers, however, and infestation can result in a measurable blood loss (anemia). The authors have seen several instances where kittens died as a result of blood loss due to heavy flea infestations. Besides itching and blood loss, fleas are a source of transmission of other diseases. The authors estimate that over 60 percent of cases of tapeworms in the cat are the result of the patient consuming tapeworm-carrying fleas. Fleas can also transmit serious bacterial diseases, such as Lyme disease (see Chapter 16, "Infectious Feline Diseases").

What Is the Treatment?

Controlling fleas on pets is a two-step process. First the environment should be treated; then the pets should be treated. The environment is that area in which fleas spend 95 percent of their time; this includes the carpeting, rugs, bedding and grass. The largest number of fleas will always be found off the pet. *There is no successful flea control program that does not involve treating the environment.*

The yard and kennel areas must also be treated thoroughly and repeatedly. Remember that rabbits, birds, squirrels and other rodents can all carry fleas and serve as a source of yard contamination. This is why these areas often need treatments year after year. Repeat treatments every month until the fleas are under control, more often in severe cases.

Because fleas do not eat often, it is less important to treat their food source, namely your pet. However, pet treatment is necessary if one is to bring the fleas under control in a timely fashion. Many different products are available for this. Shampoos, powders, oral pills, sprays, dips and collars are all used, each with its own merit. Shampoos are important in keeping the pets clean; however, they provide few long-lasting effects. Powders and sprays following a bath help provide a longer-lasting effect for about 14 days.

Dips and pour-ons are also popular, and they are very effective when applied after shampoos. Flea and tick collars are widely used as a preventative, but when used alone they do little in achieving total flea control. Fleas collars with Dursban (chlorpyrifos) are our favorite. Like all products, they work better if used in conjunction with strict environmental control.

When using any product applied directly on the pet, remember that the fleas must first get on the pets, then feed on and/or walk through the fur to become contaminated with the insecticide. They will then jump off the pet and die in the grass or carpet. It is perfectly normal to see live fleas on a pet immediately after spraying, shampooing or dipping. Many times this is confused with the products not working; however, as long as fleas are in your area you will and should expect to see them, even on the treated pet. You may continue to see live fleas for days, weeks or months, depending on the remaining flea population. The same is true with flea collars, where you can expect to see fleas directly under the collar. Again, this has to happen for the fleas to become exposed to the insecticide.

Resistance of fleas to insecticides is a topic of much discussion. Over time, all insects develop resistance, especially to mild insecticides, such as flea products. To date, it is impossible to have a product severely toxic to fleas but safe for pets, people and the environment. Flea products, for safety reasons, must be only mildly toxic, even to the fleas. The products that we select for our flea control program utilize different insecticides, such as pyrethrins, permethrins, chlorpyrifos (Dursban), and also hormone IGRs (Insect Growth Regulator). By mixing products, resistance is kept to a minimum, but still present. For tomorrow's fleas, a new product mix will be necessary. It is important to keep safety margins wide.

FELINE SCABIES (SARCOPTIC MANGE)

Feline scabies is caused by a small, microscopic mite called *Noteodres cati* (see figure 15-2). The feline scabies mite principally affects cats, but also infects dogs, rabbits and occasionally humans. It is highly contagious and therefore easily spread to cats and kittens of all ages.

The scabies mite does not spend all of its time on the surface of the skin. The male and female breed near or on the surface, but then the female eats or claws a tunnel deep into the skin, laying eggs as she goes. Her digging and waste products cause a major part of the

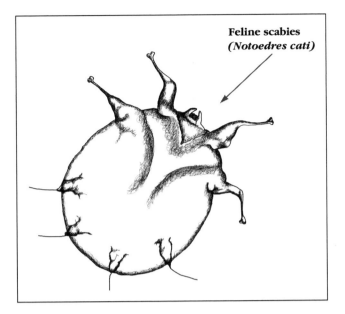

**Feline scabies
(*Notoedres cati*)**

15-2   Feline scabies

inflammation and itching sensation. After the eggs hatch, leaving more inflammatory debris behind, the larvae dig their way back to the surface, destroying more normal, healthy skin to start the whole process over again. Additionally, the various stages of the mite enjoy feeding on the host and its skin. It takes only 17 days for the entire egg-to-adult cycle to run its course before it starts over again. With this kind of reproductive capacity, one pair of mites can quickly cover an entire cat with plenty left over to colonize the next victim.

What Are the Symptoms?
Scabies in the cat has a typical pattern of distribution. It almost always begins on the head, particularly the ear regions. The mites usually infest the tips of the ears, then progress to the head, face, neck, front legs and finally the rear. Because the mites burrow into the skin, hair loss becomes evident with thick, crusty lesions developing. These areas usually cause intense itching.

What Are the Risks?
Left untreated, feline scabies can be very serious. The cat can itch so intensely and scratch so much that considerable amounts of hair fall out. The cat may be too miserable to eat, which could lead to loss of weight and finally death.

The appearance of skin lesions on the cat results from the actions of the cat more than the mite. The mite alone causes only a reddened bump or rash that is reminiscent of a mosquito bite. There will be a crusty surface in some areas formed from destroyed skin tissue. However, because of the intense itching sensation (pruritus), the cat scratches, chews and irritates the areas until this causes bleeding, scabs, hair loss, cracking of the skin and severe mutilation. As the case wears on, the damaged skin becomes thickened and the bleeding and weeping discharge is mixed with an oily seborrhea film derived from irritation of the deep oil glands.

What Is the Treatment?

Skin scrapings and mite identification with the aid of a microscope will confirm the diagnosis. Treatment is usually accomplished by clipping the remaining hair and applying an insecticidal dip. Lime sulfur is commonly used as a treatment. Various other prescription dips may be recommended and prescribed by veterinarians. It is important to treat every cat in the household; even though they may not show lesions, they may be carriers.

CHEYLETIELLOSIS—WALKING DANDRUFF

Classically, we think of this disease affecting young cats under 16 weeks of age. It is most severe in this age group (it also occurs in dogs, rabbits and humans), but all ages can be infected. There are several species of the mites belonging to the genus *Cheyletiella* (see figure 15-3). They spend almost their entire life on the host. The eggs attach to the base of the hair shafts, where they first hatch into a nymph stage, then mature into the larval form. After a week, these transform into the breeding adult and the process begins anew.

The entire egg-to-adult life cycle takes less than four weeks. The adult and juvenile stages do not burrow into the deep layers of the skin as seen with the sarcoptic mange (commonly referred to as scabies). Rather, they remain on the surface or just in the most superficial layer of the epidermis (skin). They form tunnels in the debris on the surface and draw nourishment by briefly using their heavy mouth parts to puncture the skin and suck fluids from the host's body. It is thought that cats never develop any immunity, as infestations with or without clinical signs may last for months to years.

What Are the Symptoms?

Cheyletiella infestations are usually only mildly pruritic (causing an itching sensation). Cats will scratch and chew at themselves, but usually not to the point of severe mutilation, as is common with sarcoptic mange. The areas most affected are the back (especially near the tail),

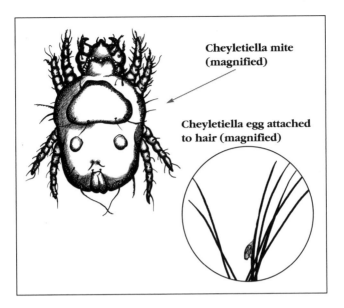

Cheyletiella mite
(magnified)

Cheyletiella egg attached
to hair (magnified)

15-3 Cheyletiella mite

the sides of the body and the head. In chronic cases, the entire coat may become involved. The affected hair coat contains scales and dandruff and will often feel oily to the touch. Patches of hair may be briefly lost, but will grow back after the mites are gone. Some adult cats can be long-term asymptomatic carriers of the mites. Their skin and coats appear perfectly normal, and they rarely scratch or bite at themselves.

What Are the Risks?
Cheyletiella mange, although not as severe as other mange, can cause intense itching. Affected animals may severely scratch and cause hair loss and raw areas of skin. Mildly infested animals may exhibit no symptoms whatsoever. It must be noted that transmissions to other animals, including humans, is not uncommon.

What Is the Treatment?
Skin scrapings to identify the mite with the aid of a microscope will yield the definitive diagnosis.

Cheyletiella infestations are easily treated with any of the milder flea and tick preparations, such as powders, shampoos, dips and/or topical sprays. We usually use flea shampoos that have either pyrethrins or carbaryl as the active ingredient. The animal should be shampooed once a week for three weeks. In severe cases, flea powder should be applied between baths. Additionally, since it has been shown that the mites can live off of the cat for up to ten days, it is best to have the home treated twice, at 14-day intervals, with insect foggers and premise sprays. *All animals must be treated even if they look and act perfectly normal.* Remember that adult cats can be asymptomatic carriers and harbor the mites for years. Not uncommonly, the owners and their families also become affected and have bites that may itch for several days or even become infected.

In our experience, many breeders and owners struggle with this disease. This happens for one of three reasons:

1. They don't treat all the animals that they have, but, rather, only those showing signs or only those closely associated with the affected ones. Remember, there will be carriers that look and act perfectly normal. These will usually be older animals, often not even part of the active breeding population. People can easily transport mites from one animal to another via their clothing.
2. They fail to treat the environment. (Remember, the mite can live off the cat for up to 10 days in the bedding, home or vehicle.) All cages, grooming tables, equipment and so on must be treated. Flea and tick kennel sprays, house sprays and foggers are all effective against Cheyletiella.
3. Catteries do not quarantine new arrivals and/or treat them preventatively before they are allowed to join the rest of the animals.

EAR MITES *(OTODECTES CYNOTIS)*

Ear mite infestation is commonly encountered in cats and kittens and diagnosed in dogs as well. Ear mites, as the name implies, are small mites that inhabit the ear canals of cats, dogs and rabbits (see figure 15-4). *Otodectes cynotis* is the scientific name assigned to the common mite of household pets, so some refer to the infestation as Otodectic Mange. In any case, a small mite is the cause and we refer to the problem as ear mites.

What Are the Symptoms?
The mites will usually cause pets to itch and scratch their ears and head. Mites feed upon the tissue lining the ear canal; their bites then causing bleeding and internal discomfort. Generally, a dark brown crust of dried blood mixed with ear wax forms inside the ear canal. The crust is easily visible and resembles coffee grounds. If your pet scratches at its ears and the ear canals appear to be filled with coffee grounds, you

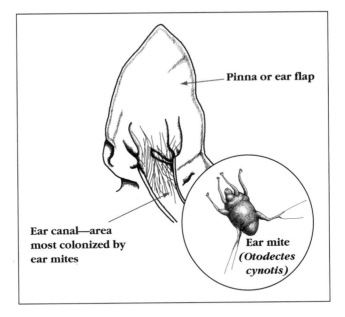

15-4   Ear mite

should suspect ear mites. One little known fact about ear mites is that they also live on areas other than the ears, such as the legs and tail.

What Are the Risks?
Ear mites will remain on the host until treated. It is very possible to have permanent or partial hearing loss as a result of a severe ear mite infestation. All suspected cases should be treated at once to avoid damage to the ear canals and/or eardrum.

What Is the Treatment?
A single mite is very tiny, almost microscopic; it's seldom noticed without the aid of a microscope. High concentrations of mites often exist on the tail, back, legs and other areas. Their presence on the body will affect the method of treatment.

Treatment is best accomplished in a two-step process. First, treat the ears and kill any mites living in them. Secondly, use an insecticidal shampoo, spray or powder to treat the rest of the animal. Destroying the mites living on other areas of the body will help prevent reinfestation of the ears. Clean the ears with an ear cleaning solution and then place ear mite drops in the ear canal daily for a period of at least seven days. Persistent cases may require treatment for a month or more. Most modern ear drops for mites contain insecticides called pyrethrins in a mineral oil base. These ear preparations are very safe and can even be used in young kittens and puppies.

The second part of the treatment involves the body and is best accomplished with an insecticidal shampoo, spray or powder designed for fleas. Excellent products are available for cats, which contain pyrethrin as an insecticide.

To recap, ear mite treatment is a two-step process:

Step 1: Place a few drops of an ear miticide into each ear daily for at least a week. Continue until the ears are clean and appear normal. This may take as long as a month.

Step 2: Treat the pet's body. We prefer to bathe the pet weekly for four weeks, using a pyrethrin shampoo. Be sure to cleanse the head, neck, body and tail areas. Once the pet is dry, use a pyrethrin spray or powder directly on the hair coat.

Unlike treating fleas, there is generally little need to treat the pet's environment. In multiple-pet households, especially those with cats, it is important to treat every pet to eliminate the transfer of mites from one pet to another. With a little effort and persistence, you can successfully treat your pet for ear mites.

TICKS

Ticks are one of the most diverse parasites affecting domestic animals, including cats. There are more than 100 species of ticks that affect birds. Another 805 species affect lizards, cattle and other animals, both wild and domestic. Although not found as commonly on cats as dogs, ticks nevertheless pose a problem to feline health.

Scientists have classified ticks into two families based upon their structure. The family Argasidae contains the soft-shelled argasid ticks. Their body lacks a hard shell (scutum), which is the protective outer covering found on some ticks. Argasids also have a ventral head and, when viewed from above, their head cannot be seen. The other tick family is named Ixodidae. These ticks possess the hard outer covering and therefore are termed hard-shelled ticks. These are the ticks that cannot be crushed between your fingers, no matter how hard you pinch.

The following is a list of the common hard-shelled (Ixodid) ticks. *Amblyomma americanum* is the Lone Star tick found throughout the South, east of the Rocky Mountains. *Amblyomma cajennense* is nicknamed the Cayenne tick and is common in Texas. *Dermacentor albipictus* is the "winter tick" and is found in the northern and western United States, as well as Canada. *Dermacentor andersoni* is the Rocky Mountain Spotted Fever tick. *Dermacentor occidentalis* is one of the most famous ticks of all. Its name is also the American dog tick, and it lives in the entire eastern two-thirds of the United States. *Ixodes scapularis* is the black-legged tick and is common on the Pacific coast. *Rhipicephalus sanguineus* is called the brown dog tick and is a serious threat to domestic animals anywhere in the United States. *Ixodes dammini* is the tiny tick known as the deer tick and the bear tick that has been documented to transmit Lyme disease to cats, dogs and humans. There are more hard-shelled ticks, but those are less frequently encountered.

The soft-shelled ticks, or Argasids, are fewer in number. The one most known is *Otobius megnini,* also known as the spinose ear tick. It is most common in the southwest and inhabits the ear canals of domestic animals.

There is no real "wood tick." Any tick that lives in brushy areas can be called a "wood tick." There is a false belief that true wood ticks exist. They do not.

All ticks have three pairs of legs during the immature stage and four pairs of legs as an adult. They crawl but cannot fly. Wings are absent. In addition, ticks possess a sensory apparatus called Haller's organ. This structure senses odor, heat, humidity and you. This is how ticks locate their food source.

Most ticks are three-host ticks, that is, during their development they feed on three different hosts (see figure 15-5). All ticks have four stages to their life cycle: egg, larvae (seed tick), nymph and adult. Adult females engorge with blood, fall off the animal and lay eggs on the ground. In one to four weeks (depending on moisture and temperature), the eggs hatch into larvae. Larvae find an animal, live off its blood for several days, then detach and fall back onto the ground. The well-fed larvae now molt into the next stage, called nymphs. The nymph finds a second animal and feeds again. Once well fed, the nymph detaches and falls back to the ground. Here it molts and changes into an adult. Both adult male and female ticks now find a third animal and once again feed on blood. Females feed for a shorter period than males. Once well fed, both males and females fall back to the ground and mate. The male now dies and the female lays eggs. Adult female ticks can live over a year. They can even survive severe winters, laying dormant under the snow. They lay the eggs in early spring, their eggs hatch and we have ticks again.

What Are the Symptoms?

The main symptom of a tick infestation is actually seeing the ticks upon the cat's body. Ticks, even the smallest, can be seen with the naked eye.

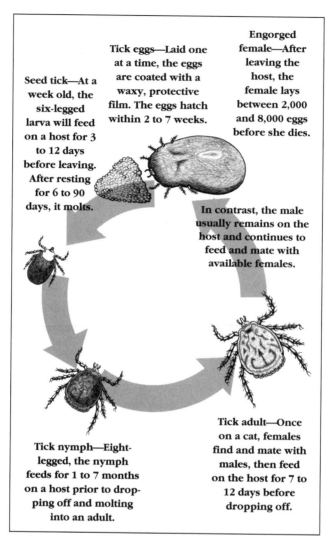

Tick eggs—Laid one at a time, the eggs are coated with a waxy, protective film. The eggs hatch within 2 to 7 weeks.

Seed tick—At a week old, the six-legged larva will feed on a host for 3 to 12 days before leaving. After resting for 6 to 90 days, it molts.

Engorged female—After leaving the host, the female lays between 2,000 and 8,000 eggs before she dies.

In contrast, the male usually remains on the host and continues to feed and mate with available females.

Tick nymph—Eight-legged, the nymph feeds for 1 to 7 months on a host prior to dropping off and molting into an adult.

Tick adult—Once on a cat, females find and mate with males, then feed on the host for 7 to 12 days before dropping off.

15-5   Typical life cycle of a three-host tick

What Are the Risks?

In addition to consuming blood, ticks are capable of spreading serious diseases, such as Lyme disease (see Chapter 16). Fortunately, most ticks do not prefer cats as opposed to dogs and other animals, so many diseases transmissible by ticks are not a serious threat to cats.

What Is the Treatment?

If only a few ticks are present upon your cat, they can be manually removed. Embedded ticks can be removed easily with tick instruments. These special devices allow one to remove the tick without squeezing the tick body. This is important, as you do not want to force harmful bacteria from the tick into the cat's bloodstream.

Once an embedded tick is manually removed, it is not uncommon for a welt and skin reaction to occur. A little hydrocortisone spray will help alleviate the irritation, but it may take a week or more to heal. Some bites may permanently scar, leaving a hairless area. Do not be worried about the tick head staying in the skin; it rarely happens. The swelling is usually due to the tick's toxic saliva, not remaining heads.

In severe infestations, it is important to treat the surrounding area, environment and the pet. Environmental tick control generally involves treating the yard and kennel areas with sprays designed to kill fleas and ticks. Spray every 30 days during the peak tick months. In northern areas, that is April through November. Remember, the cold, frosty fall weather does not kill ticks; in fact, the deer tick survives winter very well. The point here is to treat the yard late into the fall and early winter. The brown dog tick, *Rhipicephalus sanguineus,* is one of the most troublesome in yards and is found almost everywhere. Your house rarely needs treatment, as ticks do not tend to thrive in indoor areas. If you do encounter an indoor tick problem, then use a flea and tick fogger designed for fleas and other insects.

There are many different kinds of tick products to be used directly on cats. Collars, sprays and powders designed for cats are all effective at controlling ticks. Nothing prevents ticks 100 percent, but their numbers can be greatly reduced.

LICE (PEDICULOSIS)

Lice are insects that can be seen with the naked eye. They are flattened and wingless. They are very host-specific and do not tend to leave their preferred animal, in this case cats. Lice spend their entire life cycle on the pet. There are several kinds of lice, and in order to fully understand the situation, they will be identified and discussed.

Scientists divide lice into two categories: blood-sucking lice belong to the group Anoplura; those that do not suck blood, but rather chew skin, are grouped as Mallophaga.

Transmission is by direct contact with an infested pet. Unlike fleas and ticks, lice do not persist or travel in the environment. Grooming instruments may, however, serve as a source of transmission.

Lice lay eggs, or nits, on the hair shafts. The lice life cycle takes about 21 days to complete.

The most commonly encountered louse in the cat is *Felicola subrostratus* (see figure 15-6). It is a biting louse. This louse does not readily parasitize other animals, such as dogs and humans; it is specific to the cat.

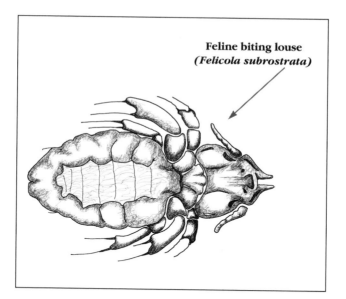

Feline biting louse
(*Felicola subrostrata*)

15-6 Feline louse

What Are the Symptoms?

The most noted sign of a louse infestation is a scruffy, dry hair coat. Hair loss may occur, and the animal may itch, at times severely so. In very heavy infestations of blood sucking lice, one may detect anemia. This is true especially in kittens. A diagnosis can usually be accomplished with the naked eye. Nits tend to be more visible than the actual louse, but both can be seen.

What Are the Risks?

Louse infestations can cause intense itching and hair loss for your pet. Kittens in particular seem to be the most affected. *Lice do not go away without treatment.*

What Is the Treatment?

Treatment is very simple. Both biting and chewing lice are easily killed with any flea and tick product. The authors prefer to bathe infected animals weekly with a pyrethrin shampoo. Once the pet is dry, dust the coat heavily with a pyrethrin flea and tick powder. Repeat this process weekly for four weeks. It usually is not necessary to treat the environment, but flea and tick foggers may help, especially in severe cases. Keep all grooming utensils clean.

Of all the parasites of cats and dogs, lice are the easiest to eliminate and they pose no threat to humans. Humans cannot get lice from animals.

CUTEREBRA FLY

The cuterebra fly larva will occasionally invade the tissues of cats and cause a boil-like skin lesion. The adult cuterebra fly lays eggs in the soil, usually in close proximity to rabbit dens. Rabbits appear to be the most common animal parasitized by the cuterebra fly. Once the eggs are laid in the soil, they hatch into small larva. These tiny, maggot-like larva climb on the fur of animals, in this case the cat, and enter natural body openings, such as the vagina, anus, urethra or nasal openings.

Once inside the body the larva migrate through the tissues to an area in the skin where they rest and grow, creating a swelling or cyst. Usually this is about the ventral neck area, but it can be anywhere on the body. Once the larva stop just under the skin, they cut a small (match head size) breathing hole through the animal's skin. The larva will grow within this skin cyst for about three weeks, then leave the animal and continue development on the ground until finally they become a mature fly, thus completing the life cycle. Fly larva in cats are usually encountered in the late summer months in the north, and slightly earlier in the south.

What Are the Symptoms?

The main symptom is a cyst under the skin. The cyst varies in size as to the age of the larva. Most "mature" larva are marble-sized. There will always be a small, easily seen breathing hole in the center of the cyst. A pink or clear serous fluid may drain from the breathing hole. Upon close examination, the larva worm can be seen through the breathing hole.

What Are the Risks?

Cuterebra larva cysts are usually not life threatening. They can be very irritating to the patient, and occasionally the skin can become infected after the larva exits. There have been cases in which the migrating larva have entered nerve tissue, such as the spinal cord, rather than becoming encapsulated below the skin. This is rare, but if it occurs, it can cause neurological damage.

What Is the Treatment?

If cuterebra larva are encountered, they can be removed by a veterinarian, usually with the aid of a forceps. Once removed, the cyst will heal.

FLY STRIKE

Fly strike refers to an infestation of maggots. This occurs as a result of maggot-producing flies laying eggs on the cat's body. This is usually the result of a skin wound or abscess serving as an attractant for flies.

What Are the Symptoms?

Maggots are easily seen in skin wounds. They resemble a small, white grub. In reality, they are simply a larval stage of several types of common flies.

What Are the Risks?

A fly strike is always serious and should be treated at once. Maggots, as they feed on the decaying tissue, excrete feces that further causes tissue destruction and death. The cat will become very ill if the tissue destruction becomes extensive.

What Is the Treatment?

All maggots should be removed or flushed from the wound. Hydrogen peroxide works well as a flushing agent. Antibiotics help treat any infections. It is especially important to clean and inspect all skin wounds, especially during the summer months when flies are the most common. Fly repellents are available for pets to help deter flies.

PARASITES OF THE HEART AND LUNGS

LUNGWORMS

The most commonly encountered parasite of the cat lungs is the lungworm, *Capillaria aerophila*. The small worm lives in the cat's lower respiratory tract. Eggs are produced that are coughed up and swallowed into the intestinal tract where they pass from the body in the feces. A cat becomes infected by ingesting eggs from fecally contaminated water or food sources and from coming in contact with egg-containing feces in litter or toilet areas.

What Are the Symptoms?

Many cats with lungworms exhibit no symptoms whatsoever. In severe infestations, however, the cat may cough or have difficulty breathing.

What Are the Risks?

Most cats either live with no harmful effects or ward off the worms naturally. In some instances, however, respiratory difficulties may become apparent. Most cases are diagnosed accidentally during routine fecal examinations for more common parasites.

What Is the Treatment?

Several drugs, including Levamisole and Fenbendazole, are effective in controlling lungworms. It is important to practice strict sanitation in households or catteries where lungworms have been problematic.

FELINE HEARTWORM DISEASE

Heartworm disease in cats is believed to be more common than previously thought. The cause is a parasitic worm called *Dirofilaria immitis*. This is the identical heartworm that commonly affects the canine. Mosquitoes are required to transmit heartworm from animal to animal.

What Are the Symptoms?
Unlike dogs, many affected cats exhibit little if any symptoms. Cats seem somewhat immune to heartworm, and affected individuals usually develop only a few adult heartworms, thus explaining the oftentimes lack of symptoms. In more severe instances, the cat may cough, experience difficulty breathing, develop heart failure and die.

What Are the Risks?
Feline heartworm disease can be fatal. In areas where heartworm is prevalent in dogs, cats should also be blood tested so that cases can be detected early.

What Is the Treatment?
There is no approved feline treatment. Ivermectin products (Heartgard feline tablets) are available to give cats on a monthly basis as a preventative.

PARASITES OF THE INTESTINAL TRACT

The majority of common internal parasites of the cat reside in the intestines. They may, at certain stages of development, occupy other areas within the body, but the adult stage is present in the intestines. Following is a discussion of those of greatest importance to cat owners.

ASCARIASIS (ROUNDWORMS)

There are basically two common roundworms in the cat: *Toxascaris leonina* and *Toxacara cati*. Their life cycles are similar, but the latter, *Toxacara cati,* is the most common. The method of infection depends on the age of the cat. Adults usually become infected by eating eggs that have been passed in the stools of cats that are carrying mature egg-laying worms. Less commonly, adult cats can become infected by eating rodents that have consumed roundworm eggs that were passed by infected cats. Kittens, on the other hand, can become infected directly from the mother while still in the uterus, immediately after birth while nursing from the mother or by ingesting the parasite eggs orally as adults do. If the eggs are ingested, once they reach the intestine they mature in one of two ways:

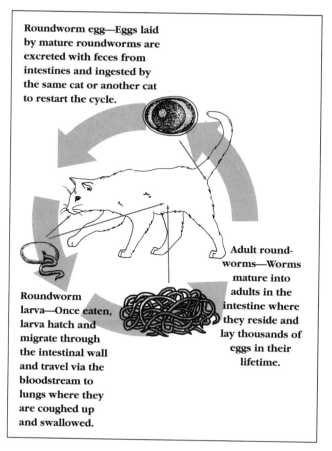

Roundworm egg—Eggs laid by mature roundworms are excreted with feces from intestines and ingested by the same cat or another cat to restart the cycle.

Roundworm larva—Once eaten, larva hatch and migrate through the intestinal wall and travel via the bloodstream to lungs where they are coughed up and swallowed.

Adult roundworms—Worms mature into adults in the intestine where they reside and lay thousands of eggs in their lifetime.

15-7 *Toxocara cati* **roundworm life cycle**

1. *Toxascaris leonina* mature within the walls of the intestine, then re-enter the cavity of the intestine and live there as adults.
2. *Toxacara cati* enter the wall of the intestine and then migrate via the lymph system to the liver and then via blood vessels to the lungs (see figure 15-7). They mature further in the lung tissue and then go up the trachea or windpipe to the throat and are swallowed, re-entering the intestine to live as adults. While in the intestine, the parasites derive all of their nutrition from the food the cat has eaten, therefore lowering the amount available to the host. If the kitten becomes infected in the uterus or while nursing from its mother, the larval worms migrate throughout the kitten's body. Some make their way to the intestine and mature to adults, while others remain encysted in the tissue and will wait to infect the next generation of kittens in the uterus or via the mother's milk.

What Are the Symptoms?

Especially in young kittens, roundworms can have devastating effects. We have all seen the pot-bellied kittens, the "poor-doers" that we blame on poor sanitation. These kittens, and many that look normal, are losing a nutritional battle to the parasites, as the worms leave little food in the intestine for the kittens to digest. By their sheer numbers the worms cause obstructions of the intestine. Through chronic irritation they often cause vomiting or diarrhea. Their migrations through the lungs can cause pneumonia. Also, the damage to the throat and trachea can cause coughing fits that can lead to further vomiting. Even the infected kittens and adults that don't show these outward signs will be less "thrifty," have poor hair coats, decreased weight gains and be more prone to other diseases.

Adult worms pass eggs into the feces and can be detected on routine fecal exams by a veterinarian. If adult worms are passed, they resemble spaghetti. Occasionally, a cat will cough up a roundworm in addition to passing them in the feces.

What Are the Risks?

As discussed under symptoms, roundworms have many effects. Although a few animals live normally with adult roundworms in their intestines, others do not. Kittens especially have a difficult time and in severe instances the kitten may die if unable to digest food.

What Is the Treatment?

Several wormers, both liquid and tablet form, are available to rid cats and kittens of roundworms. It is very important to worm kittens as a matter of routine practice. Most individuals are wormed several times over a several week period to remove all of the worms. Because the mother can easily transfer roundworms to her kittens, it is very important to worm all breeding animals routinely. At the minimum, adult cats exposed to other outdoor cats should be wormed at least twice yearly. Routine fecal exams by your veterinarian will reveal if roundworms are present. In rare instances, roundworm larva can infect humans, particularly children. In humans this is referred to as Visceral larva migrans. The worms will not reach adulthood in humans, and their main symptom is slight abdominal pain as a result of migrating larva. Humans become infected by ingesting eggs passed in cat feces. Human infestations are rare and not a matter of public health significance.

TAPEWORMS

There are several tapeworms that can affect cats and dogs, but the most common belong to either the genus *Dipylidium* or *Taenia*. *Dipylidium* is the most common cat tapeworm.

The effect of tapes on cats is usually not drastic or rapid in onset, but rather a constant drawing on available energy sources over a long period of time. Tapeworms derive their total nourishment from the same food the cat has eaten. As is often the case, however, a cat may carry several tapeworms, each several feet long. When this happens, the effects are more obvious.

For tapeworms to enter the cat's body, the cat must eat another animal that is carrying an immature stage of the parasite. For the *Taenia* tapeworm this means eating rabbits, mice, other small rodents or, rarely, small beetles. For *Dipylidium,* the cat eats fleas, and, rarely, lice that carry the larval worm. To complete the cycle, the adult tapeworm of either *Taenia* or *Dipylidium* releases small packets or segments of eggs that are passed in the feces of the cat. These are then eaten by other fleas or rodents and the whole process can start over again (see figure 15-8).

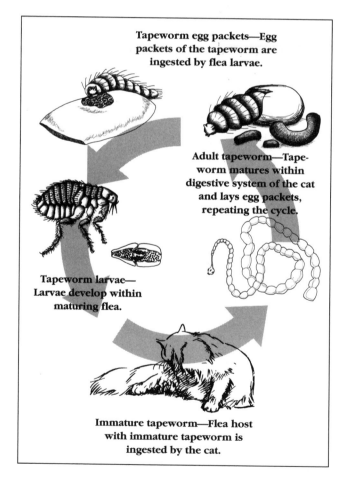

Tapeworm egg packets—Egg packets of the tapeworm are ingested by flea larvae.

Adult tapeworm—Tapeworm matures within digestive system of the cat and lays egg packets, repeating the cycle.

Tapeworm larvae—Larvae develop within maturing flea.

Immature tapeworm—Flea host with immature tapeworm is ingested by the cat.

15-8   Tapeworm life cycle

What Are the Symptoms?

Cats infested with tapeworms may appear thin, oftentimes with a poor hair coat. It must be noted, however, that many cats harboring tapeworms have no outward signs, especially if only a few tapeworms are present. A common sign is actually seeing immature worms or "segments" crawling about the anal area or in fresh stool. If the segments die and become dried to the hair, they resemble grains of rice.

Additionally, the owner can determine where a cat is getting infected. Worms of *Taenia* (from eating rodents or rabbits) have a definite square or rectangular shape, while those of *Dipylidium* (from eating fleas) are shaped more like a teardrop.

What Are the Risks?

Of all intestinal worms, tapeworms cause the least problems. Large numbers in the intestines can compete nutritionally with the cat, however, and may cause a weight loss and poor hair coat.

What Is the Treatment?

Several medications are available through veterinarians to kill tapeworms. Droncit™ is the most common wormer and is available in both an injectable and tablet form. In the case of *Dipylidium* tapeworms, strict flea control is essential in addition to worming, or the tapeworms will return in as little as 21 days.

HOOKWORMS

Hookworms that affect cats generally belong to the genus *Ancylostoma* or *Uncinaria*. They can be just as devastating as roundworms, but in a different way. Hookworms can enter the kitten while in the uterus or while it's nursing. Unique to hookworms, their eggs hatch into tiny, free-moving worms in the environment. These have the ability to penetrate directly through the skin and feet of the cat and enter its body. They go through similar migrations as do roundworms, affecting the lungs, trachea and other organs. However, the main damage we associate with them is as adults. They attach directly to the intestinal wall where they suck large quantities of blood directly from the vessels of the cat. Severe anemias develop, very often leading to death, especially in young kittens. This very large loss of blood results in the pale gums that breeders often associate with hookworm infestations. It has been estimated that an adult hookworm can consume .1 ml of blood per day. To put that in perspective, a one pound kitten only has about 40 ml of blood in its entire body. Combine this with the fact that a severely infested kitten can have hundreds of adult hookworms in its intestine. *This easily explains why death, or at least severe debilitation, results from these infections.*

What Are the Symptoms?

The most common symptom of a hookworm infestation is a loose stool, oftentimes flecked with blood. Additionally, the gums may appear pale rather than pink due to the loss of blood.

What Are the Risks?

Hookworms are severely debilitating to a cat's health. Although kittens are affected more, adult cats are at great risk too. With severe infestations, the blood loss can be so great that kittens will fail to grow at the expected rate and in some cases will die. *Hookworms must be treated at once.*

What Is the Treatment?

Hookworms are not readily identified by the naked eye. Their eggs, however, can easily be identified by routine veterinary exams of the feces. Excellent wormers are available to treat hookworms. The authors prefer pyrantel pamoate (Nemex™), which is a pleasant-tasting liquid wormer.

COCCIDIOSIS (COCCIDIA)

Coccidiosis is not a worm but rather a single-celled organism called a protozoa. The type that infects the cat usually belongs to the genus *Isospora*. They are passed in the feces of the infected individual, thereby contaminating the litter area. The other animals then ingest it orally. A typical scenario would be for the cat to walk through the contaminated area and then lick to clean the feet, resulting in the infection. It also occurs when these eggs (called oocysts in coccidia) that have been passed in the feces are ingested by mice and other rodents. If these animals are then eaten by a cat, an infection can result. Certain catteries have a recurring problem of coccidiosis affecting many but not all litters. It is believed that some adult cats are asymptomatic carriers and periodically reinfect other members of the household.

When ingested, coccidia oocysts are transported directly to the small intestine; from there they enter the wall of the intestine itself (see figure 15-9). They do not generally migrate throughout the body but remain in the wall of the intestine for their entire life. Their damage is done by directly eating and therefore destroying the lining cells of the intestine. From their home within these cells, they produce eggs that are passed in the stool of the infected cat. Severe, often bloody diarrhea is generally noted in kittens, but can be seen in cats of any age. Profuse diarrhea can result in dehydration leading to death in the young. Diagnosis can only be made by microscopic analysis of the stool. It is common to see entire litters infected. It is most common in

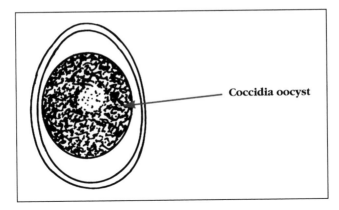

Coccidia oocyst

15-9   **Microscopic coccidia oocyst as they appear in the feces**

areas of poor sanitation, but well-kept facilities can still have a chronic problem.

What Are the Symptoms?
The most common symptom is a loose stool. Often flecks of blood or mucous will also be seen on the stool sample. If diarrhea is seen in a kitten, the number one consideration should be coccidia.

What Are the Risks?
Coccidia pose little risk to adult cats, but have a more devastating effect on kittens. It is not uncommon for kittens to die as a result of coccidia-induced diarrhea.

What Is the Treatment?
Coccidiosis is a frustrating problem to deal with when it enters a cattery. Remember, it goes directly from cat to cat as the eggs (oocysts) are passed in the stool and then orally ingested by the other cats. Drugs such as sulfadimethoxine (Albon®, Bactrovet®) are used but are not an outright killer or eliminator of coccidiosis; they only slow its growth, while the cat's immune system plays an integral part in the elimination of the organism. Additionally, it appears that there are adult cats who are asymptomatic carriers; that is, they show no signs, but can be a source from which other cats get the infection.

When a case is isolated through fecal examination, treatment is started immediately. Following the therapy, another fecal examination is done and, if coccidia are found, we extend the medication period. This will not harm the cat in any way. Usually one or two courses are enough in kittens. With adults, however, we cannot be sure as we may be dealing with a carrier where the parasites are living in a dormant state in the intestinal wall. We often put suspect carrier adults on prolonged courses of medication for 30 consecutive days. Coccidiosis is rarely a life or death matter if it is diagnosed and treated in its early stage. However, it can be a difficult problem for a cattery to eliminate completely.

GIARDIA

Giardia lamblia has long been regarded as a cause of diarrhea in humans. With an increased frequency, felines and canines are being diagnosed as suffering with giardia-induced diarrhea.

Giardia species, specifically *Giardia canis* and *Giardia cati,* are small, pear-shaped parasitic protozoa that reside within the small intestine of many animals, including domestic cats. They can only be seen with the aid of a microscope. Giardia reside naturally in streams, rivers and lakes. Additionally, any stagnant water supply such as unchanged water bowls, mud puddles, ponds, swamps and so on can all be teaming with these organisms. It is believed that wild animals, including beavers and other rodents, shed giardia in their feces, thereby contaminating the water sources. There have also been instances where giardia have been isolated in well water and municipal water supplies.

The exact mode of contamination is not always known. Most human, feline and canine cases result from drinking out of streams or lakes that may appear crystal clear yet are harboring many protozoa, including giardia. Every year there are hundreds of cases of humans who participated in outdoor recreational activities, drank directly from streams and developed this disease.

What Are the Symptoms?
A person or cat that is suffering with a giardia infestation will generally develop a severe diarrhea, usually accompanied by a fever and abdominal cramps. In the very young, very old or those debilitated by other conditions, death can result.

What Are the Risks?
Left untreated, weight loss and dehydration will be very noticeable. The fecal material from an infected individual will contain microscopic giardia cysts that will be the means of transmission. In a cattery situation, giardia can easily spread from the infected individual to many other animals. This occurs not only by water contamination, but evidence suggests that direct transmission by contact with fecal material is possible. *There is also the possibility of an owner contracting giardia directly from an infected cat.*

What Is the Treatment?

Veterinarians can only diagnose giardia by examining a fecal specimen from the patient in question. However, specialized laboratory solutions must be used to prepare the fecal sample for examination. Routine tests for worms will seldom reveal the presence of giardia organisms, as they may have become dried out and unrecognizable. Even the best giardia tests are not always 100 percent accurate in detecting the organisms. Consequently, if the diarrhea persists, the patient is treated for giardia even though the tests have been negative.

Treatment of cats suffering from giardia is accomplished with a medication known as metronidazole (trade name is Flagyl™). This drug will usually eliminate the organisms and clear the diarrhea. In chronic cases, the treatment may need to be repeated.

Prevention is aimed at providing fresh, clean drinking water and thereby reducing the cat's need to drink from other sources. There are also water filters and purifying systems made for humans available at most pharmacies. These aid in purifying stream or lake water to make it suitable for drinking. Likewise, boiling water prior to drinking may help reduce the protozoa count. In the cattery, change water daily to prevent a stagnant, contaminated water supply from developing. Lastly, in instances of severe diarrhea with no detectable cause, be suspicious of giardia.

TOXOPLASMOSIS

Toxoplasmosis is caused by the protozoal parasite, *Toxoplasma gondii.* Because it is occasionally encountered in humans with potentially devastating effects, *this is a parasite of great concern to the pet owner.*

Cats become infected with this parasite by eating infected meat. Mice are one of the main sources. Additionally, cats can acquire it by ingesting feces from an infected cat. Once infected, the cat will pass small oocysts, which are egg-like stages of the protozoa in the feces. This shedding will last two to three weeks. After the oocysts are passed in the feces, they become infective to other cats and humans in about three days. Diarrhea and fever have been reported, but most cats exhibit little if any symptoms.

Of particular concern is not the cat, but rather the humans. Humans can become infected by accidentally ingesting oocysts that were passed in the cat feces. This sounds unlikely, but it really isn't. The oocysts are microscopic and may be picked up by cleaning litter boxes or working in areas frequented by cats, such as gardens or sandboxes used as litter areas. These oocysts are not killed by soap and water and therefore can remain on "clean" human hands and become ingested during normal eating or licking of the fingers.

Most humans who ingest the oocysts have no outward effects. *Pregnant mothers are the greatest concern.* The toxoplasma organism, once inside the pregnant mother, can infect the fetus and cause permanent neurological and other damage. Prevention is the key. It is best if pregnant mothers avoid cleaning litter boxes. If this isn't possible, then rubber gloves should be worn. Pregnant mothers should also wear rubber gloves while working outside in soil, which cats may contaminate with feces. Cats belonging to pregnant women should not be allowed outdoors to hunt and should not be fed raw meat.

Although this parasite is not common, it can have devastating effects on infants. Pregnant mothers or women considering becoming pregnant should consult with their veterinarian about proper cat care during the term of the pregnancy. Toxoplasma poses little risk to the health of cats.

C H A P T E R   1 6

Infectious Feline Diseases

An infectious disease is one that is not caused by a metabolic destruction or failure of an organ, but rather an infectious agent. Bacteria, viruses and fungi are common feline pathogens that are capable of causing an infectious disease.

Infectious diseases commonly do not affect only one organ or system within the body; rather, they may affect many areas of the body simultaneously. A classic example in the cat would be feline leukemia virus. It can often affect the circulatory system, nervous system, urinary system and gastrointestinal tract simultaneously. Because of the multisystem involvement of many infectious diseases, they are usually discussed as a separate entity rather than in a chapter concerning a particular bodily system.

A discussion of infectious diseases commonly uses terminology not associated with other diseases. These terms relate to how a particular infectious agent is transmitted or spread.

Carrier is a term used to describe a cat that is harboring a disease, but otherwise appears healthy. This cat, even though it is healthy-appearing, oftentimes is capable of transmitting the infectious agent to other susceptible cats.

The **source** of the infection is a term describing whatever brings the infectious agent in contact with the cat. For instance, if the cat becomes ill from breathing a virus in the air, the air is the source. If a kitten becomes ill from a virus the mother was carrying, the mother cat is considered the source. *All infectious agents have a source.*

The **incubation period** is the time from first exposure to the infectious agent to the time the cat becomes ill. For instance, if a cat is exposed to feline distemper virus and becomes ill five days later, then the incubation period is five days.

There are literally hundreds of infectious organisms that can affect the cat. Fortunately, most are not common. Probably 90 percent of all feline infectious diseases are never encountered by a veterinarian during a lifetime of practice. Some common bacteria, viruses and fungi are a constant threat to the health of all cats everyday. It is these common and often fatal feline diseases that will be discussed in this chapter.

FELINE PANLEUKOPENIA VIRUS (FELINE DISTEMPER)

Feline distemper is one of the oldest known diseases to affect cats worldwide. However, it was not until recently (1960s) that the exact cause was identified. It is now known that the agent responsible for feline distemper is a virus, namely a *parvovirus*. Of historical significance is that in the late 1970s a parvovirus of dogs surfaced in the United States and killed literally thousands of dogs nationwide. Canine parvovirus is still a threat to dogs and probably accounts for more deaths annually than all other canine infectious diseases combined.

Of particular interest are the similarities between the parvovirus causing feline distemper and the parvovirus affecting dogs. It is common belief, though not scientifically proven, that the cats' parvovirus actually mutated and became infectious to dogs, causing the 1970s outbreak. In fact, during the late 1970s and early 1980s, the feline distemper vaccine was widely administered to dogs in hopes of stopping the spread of the canine parvovirus. It appears, from the authors' personal experiences, that during this period the feline vaccines were at least partially effective. It is also known that the feline distemper parvovirus can affect other animals including raccoons, skunks and ferrets.

Feline distemper, or more correctly feline panleukopenia, is a devastating virus to cats. It is highly contagious to all susceptible individuals. Infected cats infect others by passing stool and urine containing the parvovirus. Once eliminated from the body, the virus can live on soil, cages, litter boxes, feeding dishes, etc., for months to years.

The unaffected cat can be exposed to the virus either by direct contact with an ill cat or by picking up the virus from the environment on contaminated soil, dishes, litter boxes, etc. Once exposed, the virus incubation is short, usually about one week. The disease is severe and about 90 percent of all unvaccinated kittens less than six months old will die. Some adults may exhibit no signs of illness, but approximately 50 percent of the older, unvaccinated cats may die. It should be noted that some unvaccinated, older cats are naturally immune as they may have had prior exposure and lived, developing some immunity. In other words, some older, unvaccinated cats do carry an immunity to feline distemper.

What Are the Symptoms?

A cat with feline distemper can exhibit many signs. Kittens in particular may suffer serious effects including death. It has been well documented that the virus can infect the developing fetus while it is still in the uterus. When this happens, areas of the fetal body fail to develop properly. The most classic symptom is a condition called cerebellar hypoplasia. The **cerebellum,** the area of the brain that controls muscle coordination, fails to develop. When the kitten begins to walk (at about four weeks of age), it will move in a shaky fashion and will be unable to coordinate eating. Death will follow. In kittens exposed after birth or in adults, the most noted signs are vomiting followed by diarrhea and dehydration. The vomitus and feces might contain blood. A fever is usually present, at least in the initial stages of the disease, although later the temperature can be normal or low. Kittens and adults can die within 12 hours of exhibiting the first signs.

What Is the Treatment?

Treatment is aimed at treating the symptoms. There is no medication available to kill the specific virus. In suspected cases, veterinary advice should be sought at once. Intravenous fluids could be necessary to improve the dehydration as a result of the vomiting and diarrhea. Fortunately, excellent and safe vaccines are available to prevent this disease. Kittens should receive their initial vaccination at about six weeks of age. Boosters are usually administered at two- to four-week intervals until the kitten is 16 weeks of age, then annually for life.

FELINE RHINOTRACHEITIS VIRUS

Feline rhinotracheitis virus is suspected by the authors to be responsible for about 50 percent of all feline cases they have treated for respiratory disease. *It is generally considered to be a herpes virus.*

This disease has been known to affect cats since the 1950s. As one might suspect from a virus that principally affects the upper airways (nasal passages, trachea, larynx), it is spread through the air. A cat infected with this virus will sneeze and pass the virus into the air where it will be carried to other susceptible cats. Cats also shed the virus in saliva, tears and nasal secretions and therefore it can be transmitted to other cats by direct contact such as eating, mating or grooming. Because it is spread by the air (aerosol transmission) as well as direct contact, every patient, even those isolated in single-cat households, are at risk. The virus can persist for weeks to months under warm, moist conditions and can be carried long distances via air and air currents. Again, *every cat, even those isolated, are at risk of exposure.*

This virus is considered to be highly contagious. Upwards of 90 percent of all susceptible kittens will develop the disease if exposed. *It is also particularly contagious to cats over ten years of age.*

Once the cat is exposed, the incubation is short, usually about three days. Spread will be rapid in multiple cat households or catteries. The duration of the illness is variable, but many cats are ill for four to six weeks. Other more mildly affected cats may recover in seven to ten days. Cats who recover from this herpes virus infection will again appear normal, but are capable of carrying and transmitting this virus for up to two years. The carrier is most likely to shed the greatest number of organisms during periods of physical stress. Stress may be the result of pregnancy, surgery, parasite infestations or other diseases that can affect felines.

Infected and recovered breeding females (queens) often harbor the virus, which can cause abortions in early pregnancy. Additionally if the pregnancy goes to term, the virus lives in the vaginal tract and will infect the kittens as they are being born.

What Are the Symptoms?

The rhinotracheitis virus is similar to a severe head cold in humans. Sneezing with a nasal discharge is the most commonly noted sign. The nasal discharge may be very severe and will be yellow and thick in appearance. The eyes will also have a discharge and become crusty and difficult to open. Most cats will develop a fever, usually up to 104 degrees Fahrenheit. Occasionally a few large (pea-sized) ulcers will develop on the tongue. Ulcers of the eye, specifically the cornea, are common in kittens especially those less than six weeks of age. In severe cases the virus can attack the brain causing an encephalitis. This patient will have difficulty standing and may seizure. Kittens under six months of age and adults over ten years tend to develop the most serious infections. As a result, feline rhinotracheitis is not uncommon among cats in these age groups.

What Is the Treatment?

There is no specific medication to rid the cat of the virus. Eye ointments are used to lubricate the eyes, eliminate any complicating bacteria and reduce inflammation associated with the virus. Antihistamines are used to help decrease secretions within the airways. Antibiotics such as Amoxicillin are administered, usually orally, to prevent bacteria from also affecting the patient. Bacteria commonly try to invade stressed patients who are battling other organisms such as viruses.

To prevent this disease, all cats should be kept in well-ventilated, clean areas. Damp basements and humid conditions favor the development of respiratory diseases in cats. Fortunately, excellent and safe vaccines are available to protect cats against the feline rhinotracheitis virus. All cats and kittens over six weeks of age should remain up to date on this vaccination. Remember that your cats should be properly immunized against the feline rhinotracheitis virus.

FELINE CALICIVIRUS

Calicivirus is one of the leading causes of respiratory disease in the cat. Approximately 40 percent of respiratory infections in the feline are due to a calicivirus. Unlike many other viruses of cats, calicivirus exists in more than one strain. Since multiple strains of the virus exist, the signs and severity of a calicivirus infection vary greatly. Certain strains are more serious than others.

Regardless of strain, calicivirus attacks the cat's airways, mouth and lungs. Unlike the rhinotracheitis virus, calicivirus commonly invades deeper into the respiratory system and colonizes the lung tissue. Calicivirus does not, however, affect the eyes and nasal passages as severely as the rhinotracheitis virus does.

Once exposed, the incubation is very short. A susceptible cat may become severely ill within 48 hours of exposure. Most patients, if they survive, will recover in five to seven days. Once recovered, patients can remain carriers and shed the virus for up to a year. Additionally, the virus can persist for weeks to months in the environment. In comparison to rhinotracheitis virus, the patient with calicivirus will recover or succumb much faster. The virus is spread through the air and saliva.

What Are the Symptoms?
Symptoms vary greatly depending on the strain involved. Sneezing is common if the upper airways are involved. If the virus attacks the lungs, then coughing and difficulty in breathing may develop. Ulcers may develop on the tongue, palate and nasal areas. Unlike the rhinotracheitis virus, the eyes are not affected, so corneal ulcers are not a symptom. Because the lungs are often involved, death due to respiratory failure is common, especially in older patients and in kittens less than three weeks of age. A fever may or may not be present.

What Is the Treatment?
There are no specific medications to cure a cat of calicivirus. Oral antibiotics are used to prevent bacteria from entering the tissues damaged by the calicivirus. Medications are also administered to help dilate the bronchi and increase air flow to the lungs. Liquid or soft diets may need to be fed if the mouth ulcerations are severe and painful.

Fortunately, excellent and safe vaccines are available to protect cats and kittens over six weeks of age. These vaccines have greatly reduced the incidence of calicivirus in this century. All cats should be kept up to date throughout their entire life on calicivirus immunizations.

FELINE PNEUMONITIS (PARROT FEVER, PSITTACOSIS)

Feline pneumonitis is caused by the bacteria *Chlamydia psittaci*. During the past decade it has been increasingly recognized as a significant cause of respiratory disease in the cat. It is more prevalent than once believed. *Chlamydia,* despite its increasing prevalence, is less common and generally less severe than either feline calicivirus or feline rhinotracheitis virus. The organism is shed in the nasal secretions of infected cats and spread by direct contact. Because of the organism's large size, it is not readily spread through the air. Isolated cats and house cats are therefore at a lower risk than cats frequently exposed to others. Once exposed, the susceptible cats typically develop signs within five to ten days. The patients remain ill for several days, then recover. Relapses or flare-ups are common about two to four weeks after the patient initially recovers.

Once fully recovered, affected cats can remain carriers for up to one year, especially during periods of relapse. It is not thought, however, that normal-appearing or symptomless cats transmit the disease. Even though they harbor the organisms, they most likely only shed the organisms during a flare-up, at which time the cat will outwardly appear ill.

What Are the Symptoms?
The main symptoms of feline pneumonitis involve the nasal passages and eyes. The conjunctiva around the eyeball will appear deeply reddened and inflamed. This is usually referred to as a "meaty appearance" to the eyes. The eyeball will not be affected. A discharge is usually noted from the nostrils. *Chlamydia rarely* invades deeper within the respiratory system to reach the trachea and lungs. Because of this, neither sneezing nor coughing is common. If sneezing is present, it is usually mild.

What Is the Treatment?
Being a bacteria, *Chlamydia* responds quite well to antibiotic therapy. Tetracyclines are usually the drug of choice. Tetracycline-containing drugs are available to administer orally and into the eyes as a salve form. Usually both are used simultaneously.

Chlamydia vaccines are available and are being administered to cats with increasing popularity. Strict vaccination procedures should be followed in cats likely to be directly exposed to other cats that could possibly be harboring the disease. It should be noted that the vaccine is not totally protective. Being a bacteria, it does not stimulate as good a long-term immunity as the viral vaccines designed for feline distemper, calicivirus and rhinotracheitis. If vaccinated cats still contract the disease, they will have fewer symptoms and a quicker recovery than those who are unvaccinated.

Despite its limitations of effectiveness, modern *Chlamydia* vaccines are safe and generally recommended by veterinarians.

RABIES

Rabies is the most noted viral disease affecting domestic animals. Despite its relatively low incidence, it commands great attention because it can be spread to humans and is *always fatal once symptoms develop*. The only true test for rabies is by autopsy.

The agent responsible for rabies is a virus specifically known as rhabdovirus. It is spread from animal to animal via a bite wound as the virus is secreted into the saliva.

Many animals carry the virus and are capable of transmitting it to cats as well as other mammals, including humans. Bats, raccoons, foxes, skunks, ferrets, cats and dogs all serve as sources of the rabies virus. Rodents including mice, rats, rabbits and squirrels are not suspected of being significant sources of the rabies virus. Bats, because of their small size, are probably the most common source for a cat to encounter rabies. Bats that become ill are frequently unable to fly and fall to the grass where they easily attract the hunting cat. If the bat is harboring the rabies virus, it can easily spread it to the cat via a bite wound.

Once a rabid animal bites a cat, the incubation period is highly variable, usually between two weeks and two months. This may vary in part by the location of the bite on the cat's body. Bites about the head will generally cause the cat to become ill sooner. Once ingested into the cat by a bite wound, the virus will travel through the tissues to the nerves entering the spinal cord. From the spinal cord it moves to the brain and salivary glands where it enters the saliva and is capable of being transmitted via a bite to other susceptible animals. Once the cat becomes ill from rabies, it usually dies within eight days.

What Are the Symptoms?
There are two distinct forms of rabies in the cat. These are usually referred to as the *dumb* and the *furious* forms. The furious form is the most common. The different forms reflect the areas of nerve damage within the brain. The dumb form is exhibited as difficulty moving, progressing to paralysis and death. *The animal is not vicious.* The furious form is dramatized by a viciously attacking animal that will bite at any

object it sees. Within three to four days the rage subsides and paralysis develops, ending in death. As an owner, anytime the following neurological signs are noted, rabies should at least be considered.

Difficulty eating or swallowing, frothing at the mouth, seizures, viciousness, staggering or paralysis can all be symptoms of rabies. There are many other diseases with similar symptoms, but one must always consider rabies.

What Is the Treatment?

There is no treatment for any rabid animal; they will always die. It is absolutely essential that a cat or any animal exhibiting signs associated with rabies not be allowed to have contact with humans. If a pet exhibits the symptoms of rabies or has been in immediate contact with an animal possibly infected with rabies, then a veterinarian should be contacted at once. Your veterinarian will know the appropriate preventative measures and laws regarding rabies in your area.

Absolutely every domestic animal should receive a rabies vaccination if a vaccine has been developed for that species. Excellent and safe vaccines have been developed for dogs, cats, ferrets, cattle, horses and sheep. To date there are no commonly used vaccines for wild animals such as skunks and raccoons. Vaccinating domestic animals will lessen the likelihood of a fatal human exposure.

LYME DISEASE (BORRELIOSIS)

Most people think of Lyme as a disease affecting canines and humans. Lyme does however, affect cats with some frequency. The cause of Lyme is the bacteria *Borrelia burgdorferi*. The authors diagnosed and treated some of the first feline cases of Lyme in the state of Wisconsin. In areas where Lyme is prevalent, cats are at risk, but not with the same frequency as canines. The authors treat approximately one feline case for every 100 canine cases. Cats are usually considered more immune to Lyme than dogs. This may in part be due to their excellent grooming habits, which lessen the chances of exposure to Lyme-carrying ticks and other insects. The cat's immune system may have a greater capacity to produce antibodies against the Lyme bacteria.

As stated, Lyme disease is caused by a type of bacteria named *Borrelia burgdorferi*. Ticks, fleas, flies and other insects can carry the bacteria and are capable of transmitting the disease to susceptible animals including cats. Once exposed, the incubation period is variable, but believed to be anywhere from two weeks to several months.

What Are the Symptoms?

The cats diagnosed and treated by the authors displayed signs similar to those commonly seen in the canine. They became acutely lame in the limbs. Joint pain was evident, with several cats being almost totally unable to walk. The rear limbs seem to be the most affected, especially the knee and hip joints. Affected cats were very stiff-legged with a reluctance to move. The temperature may be normal or elevated; however, most patients have a temperature of 103 degrees Fahrenheit or more. Cats, especially those with fevers, were commonly anorexic and lethargic. Pain in multiple joints is the most characteristic sign.

What Is the Treatment?

All cats treated by the authors showed a remarkable and rapid recovery. Various antibiotics including Tetracyclines and Amoxicillin are very effective. Most patients show a marked improvement within five days of treatment; however, the treatment is usually continued for a total of four weeks to prevent relapse. At the time of this writing there is no vaccine to prevent Lyme disease in cats.

Lyme vaccines for dogs are being widely used with good success. Vaccines for cats are being studied and hopefully will be available in the future.

It is very important in the prevention of Lyme to practice strict flea and tick control. Many safe products are available for both cats and dogs. By preventing fleas and ticks, the threat of Lyme disease is greatly diminished.

FELINE INFECTIOUS PERITONITIS (FIP)

Feline infectious peritonitis (FIP) is a fairly common disease of cats. It is caused by a member of the coronavirus family. Although the disease can be seen in cats of any age, it is most commonly noted in those under five years of age. There is no difference in its incidence in males or females or between pure or mixed breed animals. Although the condition was recognized as a specific disease in the 1960s, it was not until the late 1970s that the virus was isolated and known to be the cause.

Only members of the cat family, both domestic and wild, are known to harbor the disease. It is spread directly from cat to cat. It is present in the saliva and nasal secretions of infected cats. It may, to a lesser degree, also be found in the stool and urine of these animals. Once in the environment, it is either ingested or inhaled by other cats. The organism is absorbed into the bloodstream and carried throughout the system seeding down the lymph nodes, spleen, liver and other tissues. In these areas, it usually enters specific cells that are part of the immune system referred to as macrophages.

Typically, FIP is characterized by a large buildup of fluid within the abdominal cavity of the cat (see figure 16-1). This occurs because the virus damages the walls of blood vessels and causes fluid to weep

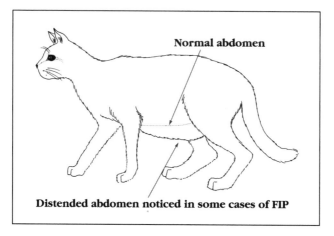

Normal abdomen

Distended abdomen noticed in some cases of FIP

16-1   Feline infectious peritonitis (FIP)

through them into the cavities of the body. This is referred to as the "wet" form of the disease. Occasionally in these cases, fluid may also develop within the chest of the infected animal. In a small percentage of those infected with the disease, no fluid is present. This is called the "dry" form of FIP.

While the fluid buildup in the abdomen or chest may affect abdominal function or respiration, it is rarely the actual cause of death. Regardless of whether a cat suffers from the wet or dry form, once clinical signs are noted, FIP is almost always fatal. The virus attacks several organ systems of the body. Clinical signs associated with FIP are similar to those of many chronic wasting diseases. These include loss of appetite, depression, weight loss, intermittent fevers and dehydration. Additionally, these animals often exhibit bleeding disorders, enlarged lymph nodes, jaundice, ocular lesions and liver and/or kidney failure. The animals also have suppressed immune systems and therefore commonly suffer from secondary bacterial infections.

As with other feline viral diseases, such as feline leukemia or feline immunodeficiency, not all cats that encounter the FIP virus react in the same way. There are at least three different scenarios that can occur. Which one occurs depends on the strength or virulence of the virus, the cat's history and the quality of its immune system.

In the first case, cats that are exposed to the virus quickly develop an effective immune response and eliminate the organism. These individuals are then immune to future FIP infections. In a second group of cats, the virus will enter their body, but be somewhat suppressed by their immune system. These cats do not eliminate the virus, but continually carry them for long periods of time—even years. It appears that the cat's immune system and the virus seem to maintain a long-term, but delicate, balance that allows them to co-exist without harm to either. These are termed "latent infections." Cats with this sort of infection carry the virus, but do not pass or shed the organism and are therefore not infectious to other animals. If cats with latent infections become sick or stressed from other diseases, their immune system often loses control over the FIP virus and they not only pass the virus to other animals, but usually develop the disease and become ill. In the final and most common possibility, the cats encounter the virus and fail to control it. It spreads throughout their bodies leading to an active infection, finally culminating in death.

Diagnosis of FIP is done through examination of the cat and its history, analysis of the fluid and specific blood tests. There are very few disorders that can cause large quantities of thick, protein-rich fluid to develop within the abdominal or chest cavity of the cat. The other possibilities can usually be eliminated from diagnosis through various diagnostic tests. The fluid present in FIP cases has certain consistent peculiarities, but is not necessarily diagnostic for this particular disease.

Cats with FIP usually produce fairly specific antibodies in response to the virus. These substances can be detected through two different types of blood tests. These are the indirect fluorescent antibodies (IFA) and the enzyme-linked immunosorbent assay (ELISA) tests. They both have the ability to detect active infections. However, these tests alone cannot be relied on in making a diagnosis as they are far from perfect. Both false-negative and false-positive results can occur. That is to say a cat testing negative may actually have the disease. In these animals, there may be no circulating antibodies. This happens frequently in the very early or the late or terminal stages of the disease.

Others may test positive, but have never encountered the FIP virus. There are several possibilities for these false-positives. This may be the result of the cat being infected with one of the FIP virus strains that is not pathogenic. That is to say that even though they make their way into the cat's body and live there for long periods of time, they are not capable of causing disease. A cat previously vaccinated with an FIP vaccine will likely test positive for antibodies. Additionally, there is a coronavirus that causes a mild intestinal infection in cats, which is referred to as **f**eline **e**nteric **c**oronavirus (FECV). It has also been shown that there are other coronaviruses that typically infect other species of animals that can also take up residence within a cat's body. Among these are the canine coronavirus (CCV) that affects dogs and transmissible gastroenteritis (TGEV) of swine. All of these related organisms make diagnosis of FIP in cats more difficult, as they all interact with current FIP blood tests and yield false-positive results.

Diagnosis of FIP is therefore usually done by the clinician utilizing all of the data available rather than just relying on a single FIP antibody blood test. In some cases, this can be very challenging, especially in the dry form of FIP or in cats that have two or more different diseases occurring simultaneously.

There is no cure for FIP. Once animals are showing clinical signs, the outcome is almost always fatal within months. With therapy some animals may go into remission, but this is not always the case. In many cases, treatment is not even recommended considering the condition of the animal, its prognosis and the potential of it being a source of infection for other animals. In those instances in which treatment is attempted, the goal can only be to slow down the progression of the disease in hopes that some immunity will develop and make the animal as comfortable as possible. To do this, the cat is treated with antibiotics to be protected from secondary bacterial infections and glucocorticoids to alter the action of the immune system. Additionally, these animals must be maintained on high quality, easily digested foods. Fluid therapy is also often necessary to maintain adequate hydration. In some cases, cytotoxic drugs such as those used in cancer therapy are also utilized. But if the cat truly has FIP, these efforts can usually only buy a brief period of time for the animal.

Today, because of the availability of a vaccine, all efforts should be taken to prevent the disease. *All cats should be inoculated on a yearly basis.* In the natural immunity against FIP, it has been found that cellular immunity is probably much more important in the protection of the cat than are circulating antibodies. This principle was taken into consideration in the formulation of the current intranasal FIP vaccine. Rather than being administered as an injection under the skin or into muscle, it is done by drops in the nose. Injectable vaccines predominately stimulate the production of circulating antibodies, which are large protein molecules that attach to and neutralize foreign invading organisms. Administration of nasal vaccine drops has been shown to stimulate the production of lines of cells that circulate through the body and have the ability to attack, ingest and neutralize infectious organisms.

FELINE LEUKEMIA VIRUS (FELV)

Today, feline leukemia virus (FeLV) is the most common cause of disease and death in cats. At one time this distinction was held by the feline distemper virus, but now the number one infectious disease is FeLV, and there is no close second. Many cat owners believe that since their animals are fairly isolated, they need not be concerned about this disorder. This is definitely not true. *The disease is responsible for over one-third of all cancer deaths in cats.* Additionally, animals die from its effects on their blood and immune systems. Others are weakened from its actions and die from unrelated secondary infections.

FeLV was discovered in 1964. The virus is believed to have developed or mutated from a virus that originally infected rats. It is classified as a retrovirus. Outside of the cat's body it cannot live for a very long time. Some experts state that it cannot exist more than 48 hours. This period is probably lengthened somewhat in areas where it remains moist. It is easily killed by most disinfectants.

FeLV is transmitted directly from cat to cat. It is passed from infected cats in their saliva and respiratory secretions. Urine and fecal passage are also possible. It can be passed from individuals licking each other, ingestion from contaminated water and food dishes or via a litter box. It is possible that it may be transmitted during sexual encounters.

Once the virus enters a cat's body, it multiplies rapidly with large numbers being present in the bloodstream within one to two months. After this point, the incubation period can vary greatly. Some animals, as we will explain later, may never develop clinical signs, while in others, symptoms can occur anytime between three months and three years.

When the feline leukemia virus enters a cat's body, the outcome is far from predictable. In a small percentage of cats, the virus will almost immediately be eliminated. The immune system of these cats responds and quickly develops an adequate level of immunity to rid the body of the organism. These cats may have had a previous exposure and were programmed to respond in this fashion, or they simply have a very effective or strong immune system. It is also possible that the strain of FeLV encountered was of low virulence or pathogenicity. Regardless, these cats will probably retain a long-term immunity against future infections.

A second group of cats, following their initial exposure to the leukemia virus, may develop what is known as a "latent" infection. In these cats, the virus does not circulate in the bloodstream and is absent from the body's secretions and excretions. It can only be found sequestered in the deeper structures of the bone marrow, spleen or lymph nodes. It may be that the immune system and the virus have reached some sort of balance that allows the virus to exist within the animal's body without either one being harmed. However, if these cats are stressed due to another illness, injury or pregnancy, the balance may be upset and the infection will transform from a latent one to an active one. The virus may then produce a clinical case of feline leukemia in the individual.

The third and most common possibility following exposure to the leukemia virus results in an active and near constant viremia (i.e., virus particles circulating through the bloodstream). This is an active infection and almost always results in a true disease syndrome. This is characterized by the virus either suppressing the immune system, actively destroying immature or developing blood cells or producing tumors.

The suppression of the immune system inhibits the cat's ability to defend itself against a wide range of infectious organisms. Many of these are relatively harmless bacteria, but in FeLV-infected cats, they can cause fatal infections.

Destruction of immature blood cells can lead to anemia if those affected are the reticulocytes, or developing red blood cells. These are the precursors of the red blood cells that are responsible for carrying oxygen throughout the body. Severe chronic or non-regenerative anemias can easily be fatal in an animal. If the precursors of the white blood cells are affected, the animal's immune system is impaired and they have difficulty defending themselves against other infectious organisms. The end result is the same as described above with suppression of the immune system. Many die from this alone.

Lastly, the virus can lead to normal cells of the lymphatic system being converted into tumor-producing cancer cells. This is referred to as lymphosarcoma. This is a progressive and fatal cancer.

The clinical signs seen with FeLV disease syndrome can vary, but it is usually characterized as a chronic wasting disease. The animal will display poor appetite, weight loss, intermittent fevers, depression, weakness and lethargy. Chronic infections of the mouth, sinuses, eyes and lungs are common. Many of these animals will have enlarged lymph nodes. Once clinical signs are noted, most of these animals will die within a few months without therapy, although some may last for two to three years. Some may undergo spontaneous remissions only to regress again, with or without apparent stress.

Diagnosis of FeLV can sometimes be made from clinical signs, history and physical examination. Most veterinarians rely on confirmation through various blood tests. There are IFA and ELISA tests to help the clinician. (See a description of these tests under FIP, earlier in this chapter.) These give positive results when they detect the presence of the virus antibodies or its antigens. However, a negative test result does not mean the cat is not infected. Most latent infections will give negative results. Therefore these tests may give less than satisfactory results when screening animals before they are brought into the home or breeding colonies. FOCMA tests are also used, which detect antibodies produced by the cat in response to the virus. These antibodies are not necessarily effective at protecting the cat, but do indicate that the animal has at least been exposed, if not infected, by FeLV in the past. Animals that are showing no signs of the disease are usually retested in six to eight weeks to see if the results have changed.

While most cats with an active FeLV infection will die, treatment can bring about a remission or at least greatly increase the comfort of the animal. These infected individuals should be recognized as potential sources of the disease for non-infected cats, and every attempt should be made to isolate them. Treatment of clinically ill cats is usually symptomatic. That is to say that the clinician attempts to support the animal, increasing its resistance to secondary infections and suppressing the disease processes as much as possible.

Treatment regimes generally include broad spectrum antibiotics, glucocorticoids (cortisones), fluids, concentrated nutritional supplements and, in some cases, chemotherapeutic agents that attack cancer cells. These efforts will rarely, if ever, cure the animal, but they may significantly lengthen its life.

Today, vaccines are available that provide excellent protection against FeLV. It is important that cats be vaccinated before they are exposed to FeLV as animals that already carry the virus will derive few if any benefits from the vaccine. Some believe that vaccination may stimulate the immune system of some animals with latent infections, enabling them to eliminate the virus from their bodies. At the present time there is little research to support this theory. All cats should be inoculated on a yearly basis throughout their lives.

Often owners with multiple-cat households only vaccinate those animals who go outside or travel to shows or boarding facilities. This can result in disaster for their other non-vaccinated animals. While vaccinations will protect a cat from the disease, following exposure to FeLV, these animals may briefly carry the virus in their body and later shed it. In this way, immune protected animals can carry the virus home to other cats.

FELINE IMMUNODEFICIENCY VIRUS (FELINE AIDS OR FIV)

Feline immunodeficiency virus (FIV) is the feline counterpart to the human AIDS virus. While it is different and cross infection between humans and cats does not occur with FIV, the two diseases parallel each other almost exactly. FIV was first isolated and understood to cause this disease in 1986. It is in the **retrovirus** group. Specifically it belongs to the *lentivirus* subfamily.

Although FIV can be found in the blood and numerous tissues of the body, some of the highest concentrations are present in the saliva of infected cats. It is usually transmitted from cat to cat through bite wounds. All domestic cats can potentially become infected, but because of the method of transmission, it is most common in free-roaming male cats frequently fighting to defend their territory or during breeding periods. It can occur in multi-cat households and catteries, but its incidence is generally much lower in these situations. Cats showing clinical signs of the disease are generally older due to the pro-longed incubation period following exposure.

Once the virus enters the body of a cat, *it may be years before any significant clinical signs are noted*. This characteristic and the progres-sion of the disease within the cat's body closely parallel the pattern of the human AIDS virus. After the initial exposure, the virus spreads through the affected animal's body infecting a wide range of cells. Many different types of cells of the immune system quickly become involved. Illustrating the ability of the virus to enter many different tis-sue types is the fact that it can be isolated during these early stages in the nervous tissue of the brain and numerous cell types within the gas-trointestinal tract. In these first few months the only outward signs observed would be mild diarrhea and lethargy.

Infected animals then enter into a potentially long dormant (qui-escent) period with few clinical signs. During this time, which usually lasts several years, the virus continues to multiply, affecting more and more cells.

When the first clinical signs do appear, they certainly are not specifi-cally indicative of FIV. These cats will show poor appetites, weight loss, intermittent fevers, depressed numbers of various white blood cells and an overall poor appearance. Some may show signs resulting from the infection of the nervous tissue varying from an abnormal gait, twitching of facial muscles and back and forth movement of the eyes, to aggression or partial paralysis.

As the condition worsens, most systems of the body become involved. This can be the result of secondary infections due to the sup-pression of the cat's immune system or to the direct action of the virus on the animal's tissues. Inflammations and infections commonly occur within the eyes, mouth, lungs, skin and gastrointestinal tract. In some of these animals it appears that all areas of their bodies are going through some form of spontaneous breakdown. Additionally, infections spread easily throughout the body doing much more damage than would normally be expected.

Diagnosis is often complicated and FIV can easily be confused with other conditions, such as FIP and FeLV. These cats will have lower-than-normal numbers of most types of white blood cells. Additionally, production of new cells will be retarded or non-existent. The red blood cells will be decreased in number, classifying the animals as anemic. Tumors of the lymph nodes are not uncommon.

Although the specific blood tests used to detect FIV are not perfect, they are heavily relied on at this point for a diagnosis. Those most commonly utilized by diagnostic clinicians are the indirect immunofluorescent antibody (IFA), enzyme-linked immunosorbent assay (ELISA) and the Western blot test. False-negative results sometimes occur in the very early or very late stages of the disease. False-positive results can also occur, but they are less common.

What Is the Treatment?

Treatment can be attempted in FIV-infected cats, but once they reach a stage with outward clinical signs, the prognosis is very poor. Most of these animals will die within eight months. When treatment is attempted, it consists of broad spectrum antibiotics to protect the animals against secondary bacterial infections, glucocorticoids (cortisones) to decrease adverse immunological problems, easily digested high quality nutritional supplements and fluid therapy to offset dehydration if present. Severely anemic patients are sometimes given blood transfusions. The glucocorticoids are also useful because they have a euphoric affect on the patient that increases their desire to eat and drink.

No vaccination for FIV exists at this time. Since the disease is spread primarily through bite wounds, non-infected cats can be protected by preventing direct contact with other cats. Individuals may choose to test new animals before they are brought onto their premises.

RINGWORM

Ringworm, also referred to as dermatophytosis, is a specific skin disease caused by fungal organisms. The disease gets its name from the circular lesions that usually occur. Despite the name ringworm, it is not a worm but rather a fungus. The term is often used incorrectly to describe a wide range of dermatological disorders. In the cat, most cases of ringworm are caused by either *Microsporum canis* or *Microsporum gypseum*. These same fungal organisms can cause ringworm in a wide range of species, including humans.

In the cat, ringworm usually spreads from animal to animal through direct contact. It can also be spread through contact with contaminated bedding, cages, furniture or food dishes. All of the fungal organisms responsible for this disease in the cat form resistant, resting spores that can live freely in the environment for extremely long periods of time. They are normal inhabitants of soil. Additionally, these organisms can be routinely cultured from the skin and coats of normal cats that show no signs of the disease. Many cats are thought to be asymptomatic carriers, harboring the organisms their entire lives without ever actually exhibiting signs of the disease.

Regardless of where the animal contracts the fungal organism, the course of the disease is quite similar. It primarily involves the hair follicle and the hair itself. The fungi enter the hair follicle, colonize it and attach to the surface of the developing hair shaft. They cause the hair to become brittle and it breaks apart. The skin cells surrounding the follicle can also become involved. As the hair and skin cells die, they fall from the animal and carry fungal organisms and their infectious spores to other animals.

In the cat, the lesions produced by ringworm can vary greatly. Classically, these are the dry, scaly circular lesions showing a nearly total loss of hair. They range in color from gray to brown. They can occur anywhere on the cat, but are most often seen near or on the head. The cats rarely scratch. Rather the lesions seem to spontaneously arise and grow to one-half to two inches in diameter. The hair falls away leaving only a thick, crusty lesion whose surface continually flakes off. Some animals will develop areas of hair loss, but the surface of the skin will be moist and weep a clear to pinkish fluid rather than be crusty.

In some cats, raised hairless nodules or masses will occur. These are usually 1/4 to 1/2 inch in diameter. This condition is referred to as granulatous dermatitis. These lesions can also appear anywhere, but are frequently seen on the face and legs.

In other cats, no distinct lesions are noted. Rather there is a generalized loss of hair over wide areas of the body. Additionally, many cats with ringworm develop infected toenails as a result of the fungus invading the nail beds. These have a crusty buildup where they meet the skin and the nails become deformed in appearance. In some cats, they break off easily.

Not all cats are equally susceptible to ringworm infections. As previously stated, many carry the fungal organism all of their lives and never show any lesions. Whether a cat becomes clinically infected is believed to be determined by the individual animal's immune system. Those cats with immune systems that respond to the fungi do not develop lesions, but simply carry the fungus on their body. Often cats with diseases that suppress the immune system, such as feline leukemia or feline infectious peritonitis, have secondary fungal infections of the skin. The use of drugs such as steroids, which in high doses may inhibit the immune response of cats, may make them more sensitive to fungal infections. Additionally, long-haired cats seem to be more prone to the disease, especially Persians and Himalayans. Kittens are always more susceptible than adults, probably because their immune systems are not fully developed.

Diagnosis can usually not be made by the appearance of the lesions alone. This is usually accomplished through the microscopic examination of hair shafts and actually seeing the fungal organisms or by culturing infected hairs and dander. Cats can also be examined with the use of a Wood's light. When this black light tool is held over a cat's hair coat, areas infected with the fungus *Microsporum canis* will fluoresce a bright green color. This test is specific for *Microsporum canis* as other types of fungal organisms do not fluoresce.

Treatment is directed both at the infected animal and the animal's environment. The hair surrounding the lesions is usually clipped and topical treatments of antifungal creams, lime-sulfur rinses and iodine chlorhexidine shampoos are used on a routine basis. Usually more than one topical preparation is used. In more severe cases, oral medications are also used. In the past, griseofulvin was the drug of choice, but today many veterinarians prefer the newer and more rapid-acting keto-conazole or some of its derivatives. Ketoconazole is also safer than griseofulvin, because it produces fewer side effects in cats.

Because the cat's surroundings become contaminated with infectious fungal spores, the environment must also be treated. Dishes, bedding, cages, floors and even carpeting should be disinfected. Chemical disin-fectants can be used on hard surfaces; bedding should either be dis-posed of or washed in bleach solutions. Carpet and furniture can be steam-cleaned. Not every case requires all of these things be done, but in multi-cat households where several animals are infected it will prob-ably be necessary to truly control the situation.

A vaccine is available today that can be used as both a preventative and as part of a treatment scheme. In many catteries, the vaccine has been found to be almost indispensable in eliminating the disease from the premises.

FELINE INFECTIOUS ANEMIA (HAEMOBARTONELLOSIS, FIA)

Feline infectious anemia (FIA) is a cause of anemia in cats throughout the world. The agent involved is a rickettsial bacterial organism that invades and destroys red blood cells, causing the anemia. It is not known exactly how it is spread from cat to cat. It can, however, be transmitted through the uterus to the unborn fetus. Bite wounds are also a suspected method of transmission. Fleas and other insects are probably carriers. Male cats show a higher incidence of infections than females.

What Are the Symptoms?

Infected cats will be depressed and usually have a fever. Although some carrier cats may *appear* normal, most lose weight and have poor appetites. As the red blood cells are destroyed by this parasite, the red pigment is released from the dead cells, creating jaundice. Jaundice is yellow-appearing skin and eyes as a result of the released red blood cell pigment.

What Are the Risks?

Feline infectious anemia can be fatal. Some cats live fairly normal lives; however, periods of stress will cause the parasite to multiply and worsen the cat's condition.

What Is the Treatment?

If the cat is severely anemic, blood transfusions may be necessary to replace the destroyed red blood cells. Various drugs including Oxytetracycline have been successfully used in treating this parasite.

FADING KITTEN SYNDROME

This condition, also referred to as kitten mortality complex, describes the effect of a wide range of organisms on newborn kittens. During the first few days of life, individual kittens or entire litters can become ill for no apparent reason and slowly die.

The signs associated with this syndrome can vary greatly. In some cases, the females fail to become pregnant or their kittens die while still in the uterus. These kittens may be reabsorbed by the mother, aborted or born dead. Typically, however, the kittens are alive at birth and nurse normally for a day or two, but suddenly discontinue feeding, vocalize as if hungry or in pain, develop swollen, gas-filled abdomens, may have diarrhea, show a drop in body temperature and finally will die.

While there is no single causative agent, most cases are believed to be brought on by various bacterial or viral organisms. Those often isolated are the feline infectious peritonitis virus, feline leukemia virus and a wide range of bacterial species.

While there is no treatment for the viral agents, kittens affected with bacteria can be safely treated with antibiotics. The mother should also be treated. Additionally, these kittens will need to be kept warm and given fluids and nutritional supplementation. It is very important that signs be recognized early and treatment started as soon as possible. Even with heroic efforts, a significant portion of these animals may die.

Animals associated with these kittens, either their mother or house-mates, should be tested for the various viral diseases, including FIA, FeLV and FIV. Those showing positive results should not be bred and should be removed from the premises in catteries. As a preventative, queens may be placed on antibiotics such as Amoxicillin during the last week of pregnancy and the first week of nursing. This will help protect the kittens against bacterial diseases and cause them no harm.

Feline Facts

A P P E N D I X   A

NORMAL PHYSIOLOGICAL DATA FOR THE FELINE

Average Body Temperature................................101.5 degrees Fahrenheit

Average Pulse (Heart Rate).......................................120 beats per minute

Average Respiratory Rate..25 breaths per minute

Average Gestation...63 days

ROLE OF ASH IN THE DIET

Frequently when discussing feline nutrition and related disorders, such as feline urological syndrome (FUS, see page 194), the term ash is used.

Ash is one of the most misunderstood components of a diet. All foods, including those of humans, contain ash. We would die or be very ill without it; the same is true of our pets.

Dietary ash is defined in this matter. When a food sample is burned at 1,112 degrees Fahrenheit for two hours, the residue that is left is termed "ash."

Ash is absolutely necessary in a diet because it contains all the essential minerals, such as calcium, phosphorous, salt, iron, magnesium, etc. These minerals are needed for normal bodily functions.

Different foods contain varying levels of ash. In general, canned foods contain less ash than dry foods. This is because canned foods contain more moisture than dry foods and, therefore, contain a lower percentage of ash.

The amount of ash is generally not listed on the food bag analysis. Ash is adequate in all name-brand commercial foods and is usually around 8 percent in dry foods and 3.5 percent in canned foods.

Occasionally veterinarians will place dogs and cats on a restricted ash diet. This is generally done to pets that have a tendency to develop bladder stones. The role of dietary ash in these patients is unclear, but a low ash (less than 1.4 percent), is oftentimes suggested. The feeling here is that since many times the bladder stones are composed of magnesium, calcium and phosphorus, then by restricting the dietary intake of these minerals, we may be able to discourage future bladder stone formation.

FELINE MEDICATIONS,
USES AND COMMON DOSAGES

Common Drug Name	Use	Dosage
Acetylsalicylic Acid (Aspirin)		Not recommended
Amoxicillin	Antibiotic	10 mg per pound, every 12 hours, orally
Amoxicillin plus Clavulanate (Clavamox)	Antibiotic	62.5 mg, every 12 hours, orally
Cefadroxil (Cefa-Drops)	Antibiotic	11 mg, per pound, every 24 hours, orally
Dimenhydrinate (Dramamine)	Motion sickness	12.5 mg, every 8 hours, orally
Diphenhydramine Hydrochloride (Benadryl)	Antihistamine helps allergies	up to 2 mg per pound, every 8 hours, orally
Kaolin/Pectin (Kaopectate)	Anti-diarrheal	1 ml per pound, every 4 hours, orally
Ketoconazole (Nizoral)	Antifungal (Ringworm)	5 mg per pound of body weight, every 12 hours, orally
Metronidazole (Flagyl)	Giardia and Colitis	5 mg per pound, every 12 hours for 5 days, orally

Oxytetracycline	Antibiotic	10 mg per pound, every 8 hours, orally
Pyrantel Pamoate (Nemex)	Wormer	10 mg per pound, orally, repeat in 2 weeks
Sulfadimethoxine (Albon, Bactrovet)	Coccidia	12 mg per pound, every 24 hours for 3-7 days, orally

Note—In treating certain or specific diseases, veterinarians may alter the dosages from those listed. On these and all medications, always follow the advice of your veterinarian.

Glossary

Abscess—A pocket of infection filled with white blood cells.

Acne—A disorder of the skin characterized by the formation of pustules.

Acute—Of short and quick recourse. An acute illness is generally of rapid onset.

Allergen—A substance capable of triggering an allergic response. Examples are flea saliva and pollens.

Alopecia—A loss of hair or baldness.

Amino Acid—Organic compounds used to build proteins. Taurine is a noted example in the cat.

Anemia—A condition resulting from abnormally low numbers of red blood cells.

Angiogram—A study of the blood vessels and heart by placing dye into the bloodstream and tracking its movement, usually via radiographs (X-rays).

Antibiotic—A drug used to treat bacterial infections.

Anticonvulsant—A drug used to prevent or decrease the severity of convulsions.

Antihistamine—A drug used to suppress the release of histamine as a result of an allergic response.

Anti-inflammatory—A drug that suppresses inflammation. Cortisone is one of the best known examples. Newer anti-inflammatory drugs approved for use in dogs, have not been approved for cats to date.

Arthritis—Sometimes referred to as osteoarthritis, an inflammation of a joint.

Articulation—A joint between two bones.

Asthma—Difficulty breathing as a result of constrictions of the airways, usually as a result of an allergic response.

Asymptomatic—A term used to describe a condition in which no symptoms are present.

Autoimmune—A condition in which the body destroys its own cells.

Benign—A non-severe condition not likely to spread or invade into other areas of the body.

Carrier—An animal that is harboring a disease and is capable of transmitting it to others.

Cattery—A term used to describe an area where breeding cats are kept.

Chemotherapy—The use of chemicals to treat certain diseases.

Chronic—Of long term. A chronic illness is one of long duration.

Congenital—A condition that exists at birth.

Cortisone—A type of steroid used to decrease inflammation.

Cyanosis—A blue or gray appearance of the tongue, gums and skin as a result of an oxygen deficiency.

Cyst—A fluid-filled sac or swelling within the tissues.

Debilitation—A loss of strength.

Dermatitis—An inflammation of the skin.

Diuretic—A drug used to increase urine production and remove excess fluid from the body.

Dystocia—A labored birthing process.

Dystrophy—An abnormality in development.

Eczyma—A term used to describe an inflammation of the outer skin layers. Usually characterized by scaling, redness and itching.

Edema—An abnormal accumulation of fluid within the cells, commonly the cause of swelling following trauma.

EKG—Electrocardiogram, used to measure the electrical conduction within the heart muscle.

Epilepsy—A medical condition characterized by seizures.

Epiphora—An overflow of tears upon the cheeks due to a blockage or narrowing of the tear ducts.

Foreign Body—Any abnormal substance. A splinter is an example of a foreign body of the skin.

Fracture—A break or crack in something hard, such as bones or teeth.

Granuloma—The formation of a nodule as a result of inflammation.

Hematoma—A mass of blood within the tissues. Generally the result of trauma to the blood vessels or abnormal blood clotting.

Hernia—The protrusion of tissue through the structures that normally contain it.

Hormone—A chemical substance produced by one organ and carried by the bloodstream to affect another organ.

Hyperplasia—An increase of the number of cells within an organ.

Hypersensitivity—A severe or abnormally high reaction to an allergen.

Hypoplasia—An underdevelopment of an organ or tissues.

Immunization—Synonymous with a vaccination. If a cat is vaccinated then it is said to be "immunized."

Inherited—A trait passed from one generation to the next.

Jaundice—Sometimes referred to as icterus; a yellowing of the skin and eyes, usually as a result of a liver or red blood cell disorder.

Kindling—A term occasionally used to describe the act of giving birth to kittens.

Latent—A dormant stage of a disease; the patient is infected with an organism, but is not yet ill.

Lethargy—To be without energy almost to the state of unconsciousness; to feel drowsy.

Leukemia—A lower-than-normal level of white blood cells within the blood.

Luxation—A term used to describe a dislocation from a normal position.

Magnesium—A chemical element found in all foods that may be linked to certain disorders, such as the development of bladder stones.

Malignant—An invasive disorder likely to cause death.

Mange—Any of several skin and ear conditions caused by a variety of mites.

Metabolism—The process of energy utilization by the cells.

Ovulation—The release of an egg from the ovary of the female.

Parasite—An organism that lives upon or within another and feeds upon it.

pH—A term used to describe the acidity or alkalinity of a substance such as urine.

Pneumonia—Fluid buildup within the lungs.

Polydactyly—The presence of extra toes.

Polyp—A small growth from mucous membranes such as those lining the nasal cavity and intestinal tract.

Queen—An unspayed female cat used for breeding.

Regurgitation—The backward flow of material; commonly used to describe the expelling of food.

Ringworm—A condition resulting from a fungus. The circular appearance of a fungus lesion resembling a worm. However, ringworm is not a worm.

Sclerosis—A hardening of tissue, usually the result of chronic inflammation.

Seborrhea—An abnormal secretion of oils from the skin glands.

Seizure—An attack or sudden onset of symptoms; generally related to the nervous system of individuals affected with epilepsy.

Starch—A storage form of sugars (carbohydrates); may react with water to create various forms of sugars.

Symptom—A term used to describe a deviation from normal. If something is not normal in appearance, function or sensation, then it may be described as a symptom.

Tomcat—An unneutered male cat.

Ulcer—A lesion in which the tissue surface is eroded away.

Index

Abscessed tooth roots, 26–27
Abscesses
    retrobulbar, 144–45
    skin, 172–73
Acne, feline, 169–70
Acute renal disease, 186–87
Adam's apple, 74
Addison's disease, 101–2
Adenocarcinomas, 58, 59, 82
Adenoma, 102, 103
ADH (anti-diuretic
    hormone), 104
Adrenal glands, 97
    disorders of, 100–102
Adrenaline (epinephrine),
    100
Adrenal sex steroids, 97–98
Adrenocorticotropic hor-
    mone (ACTH), 97
AIDS, feline (feline immun-
    odeficiency virus), 241–43
Albinism, 153
Aldosterone, 100
Allergic dermatitis, 168–69
Allergies
    conjunctivitis due to,
      134, 135
    to fleas, 165
    food, 168, 169
    inhalation, 168
Alopecia (hair loss or
    baldness)
    facial, 167–68
    feline endocrine, 104–5
    psychogenic (neuro-
      dermatitis), 164
Alveoli, 70–71
American dog tick, 211
Androgens, 100
Anemia, feline infectious
    (FIA), 245–46
Anestrus, 4
Anisocoria, 120
Antibodies, 197

Anti-diuretic hormone
    (ADH), 104
Antigens, 197
Anus, 66
Aortic stenosis, 94
Arterial thromboembolism
    (saddle thrombi), 88–90
Arthritis (osteoarthritis), 108,
    112–13
Ascariasis (roundworms),
    217–19
Aspirin, 113
Asthma, bronchial, 83–84
Atria of the heart, 85
Atrioventricular valve
    complex malformation, 90
Auricular hematoma,
    177–78
Autonomic nervous system
    (ANS), 119
Azotemia, 187

Bad breath, 34, 36
Balance (equilibrium), 175
Baldness. See Alopecia
Basal cell tumors, 166
Bile, 41, 42, 46, 47
Bile acids, 41
Bile duct, 41
Bilirubin, 41
Blackheads, 169–70
Bladder, 185
    cystitis, 190–91
Bladder stones, 103
Blindness, 138, 140, 148,
    151, 152, 155, 158
Blood loss (anemia), fleas
    and, 203
Bone and joint disorders,
    108–15
    fractures, 113–15
    luxated patellas,
      111–12
    osteoarthritis, 112–13

polydactylism, 111
tumors, 115
Bones, 107. See also Bone
    and joint disorders; Muscu-
    loskeletal system
Borreliosis (Lyme disease),
    234–35
Brain
    cerebellar hypoplasia,
      126–27
    hydrocephaly, 122–23
    infections, 125–26
    injury to, 119–21
    tumors, 121–22
Breathing. See Respiratory
    system
Breeding, 4
Bronchial asthma, 83–84
Brown dog tick, 211

Calcitonin, 102
Calcium, 185–86
    primary hyperparathy-
      roidism and, 103
Calicivirus, feline, 134, 135,
    231–32
Cancer. See Tumors
Cardiac sphincter, 52
Cardiomyopathy, 86–88
Carrier, defined, 227
Cataracts, 157–58
Cavities (caries), 25–26
Cayenne tick, 210
Cecum, 66
Central nervous system
    (CNS), 119. See also Brain;
    Spinal cord
Cerebellar hypoplasia,
    126–27
Cerumen glands (lubricating
    glands), cancer of, 167
Chest wounds, 80
Cheyletiellosis (walking dan-
    druff), 206–8

Chlamydia psittaci, 134, 135, 232–33
Chronic endometritis, 8–9
Chronic renal disease, 187–88
Chymotrypsin, 43
Cilia, 71
Circling, 120
Circulatory system, 85–95. *See also* Heart and circulatory diseases
anatomy of, 85
Cleft palate, 33–34
Closed fractures, 113
Coccidiosis (coccidia), 222–24
Colitis, 66
Collars, fleas, 204
Colon, 66. *See also* Large intestine
Compound fractures, 113
Congenital megaesophagus, 49–51
Congestive cardiomyopathy, 86
Conjunctiva, 132, 133
Conjunctivitis, 133–35
Constipation, 67, 68
Convulsions, 120
Cornea, 129
entropion and, 138
foreign bodies in, 145–47
prominent nasal folds and, 141–42
trauma to, 149–50
Corneal dystrophy, hereditary, 150
Corneal sequestration, 148–49
Corneal ulcers, 138, 140, 146–48
Coronaviruses, 237
Corticosteroids, 97, 100
Cortisol (hydrocortisone), 100
Cortisones, 98
Coughing
in asthma, 84
tracheobronchitis and, 77
Cruciate ligament (knee joint), ruptured, 115–16

Cryptorchidism, 20
Crystals, urinary, 194
Cushing's disease (or syndrome), 100
Cuterebra fly, 215
Cystic endometrial hyperplasia, 8
Cystitis, 5, 190–91
Cysts
cuterebra larva, 215
in inherited polycystic kidney disease, 188–89
iris, 152
meibomian, 136, 137
ovarian, 5–6

Dandruff, walking (cheyletiellosis), 206–8
Deafness
aging and, 183
hereditary, 183
Deciduous teeth, 23–25
Deer tick, 211
Dehydration, 187
Dental caries, 25–26
Dermatitis
allergic, 168–69
flea bite, 165
miliary, 163
solar, 166
Dermatological disorders. *See* Skin disorders
Dermis, 161
Detached retina, 154–55
Diabetes insipidus, 104
Diabetes mellitus, 98–99
Diabetic cataracts, 157, 158
Diaphragm, 70
Diaphragmatic hernias, 81–82
Diarrhea, small intestine disorders and, 59–60, 65
Diet
constipation and, 67
gingivitis and, 32
Digestive tract, 49–69
Disc, herniated (slipped or ruptured disc), 116–18
Distemper, feline (feline panleukopenia virus), 228–29

Drooling, 35
excessive (ptyalism), 37–38
Ductus arteriosus, 90
patent (PDA), 91–93
Duodenum, 53, 59
Dystocia, 12–13

Ear canal, 175
foreign bodies in, 182
infections of (otitis externa), 178–79
Ear disorders, 175–83
auricular hematoma, 177
deafness, 183
foreign bodies in the ear canal, 182
infections of the middle ear (otitis media), 181–82
infections of the outer ear (otitis externa), 178–79
parasites of the outer ear (ear mites), 179–81
Eardrum, 175
Ear flaps (pinna), 175, 177
Ear mites, 179–81, 200, 208–10
Ears. *See also* Parasites, of the skin and ears
cleaning, 179
Eating foreign objects (PICA), 34–35
Eclampsia (lactational tetany or milk fever), 18–19
Ectoparasites, 200
Ectopic pregnancy, 11–12
Ectropion, 138–39
Ejaculation, 2
Encephalitis, 125
Endocarditis, vegetative, 88
Endocrine alopecia, feline, 104–5
Endocrine glands, 97
Endometrial hyperplasia, cystic, 8
Endometritis, chronic, 8–9
Endoparasites, 200
Enteritis, 59, 60
parasitic, 64–65

Entropion, 137–38
Eosinophilic granuloma
    complex, 171–72
Eosinophilic plaque, 171
Epidermis, 161
Epiglottis, 74
Epilepsy (seizures), 123
Epinephrine (adrenaline),
    100
Epiphora (tear staining), 143
Epiphysial fractures, 113
Equilibrium (balance), 175
Erythropoietin, 186
Esophagus, disorders of,
    49–52
Estrogens, 1, 6, 10, 97, 100
Estrous heat cycle, 3–4
Estrus, 4
Eyeball
        disorders of, 145–50
        retrobulbar abscess
            behind, 144–45
Eye chambers, disorders of,
    150–52
Eyelashes, 132–33
Eyelids, 132–33. See also
    Third eyelid (nictitating
    membrane)
        ectropion (everted
            lower eyelids),
            138–39
        entropion (inverted
            eyelids), 137–38
        meibomian gland infec-
            tions, 136–37
Eyes, 129–59
        anatomy of, 129–30

Facial alopecia, 167–68
Fading kitten syndrome,
    246–47
Fatty liver disease (hepatic
    lipidosis), 44–45
Feline endocrine alopecia,
    104–5
Feline enteric coronavirus
    (FECV), 237
Feline immunodeficiency
    virus (feline AIDS or FIV),
    241–43
Feline infectious anemia
    (FIA), 245–46

Feline infectious peritonitis
    (FIP), 46, 125, 235–38
Feline leukemia virus
    (FeLV), 125, 197, 199,
    238–41
Feline panleukopenia virus
    (feline distemper), 228–29
Feline pneumonitis (parrot
    fever, psittacosis), 232–33
Feline rhinotracheitis virus,
    229–31
Feline scabies (sarcoptic
    mange), 204–6
Feline tail gland hyperplasia
    (stud tail), 162–63
Feline urological syndrome
    (FUS), 194–96
Female reproductive system,
    1–19
Fetal membranes (retained
    placentas), 14–15
FIA (feline infectious ane-
    mia), 245–46
Fibrosarcomas, 167
Flea and tick collars, 204
Fleas, 64, 200–204
        controlling, 203–4
        hypersensitivity to,
            165
        resistance to insecti-
            cides, 204
        types of, 201
Fly strike, 215–16
Follicle stimulating hormone
    (FSH), 97
Food allergies, 168, 169
Foreign bodies
        behind third eyelid,
            140–41
        in cornea, 145–47
        in the ear canal, 182
        in the esophagus, 52
        in mouth, 35–36
        in nose, 73–74
        in the small intestine,
            62–64
        in the stomach,
            56–57
Fractures, 113–15
Frostbite, 173–74
FUS (feline urological syn-
    drome), 194–96

Gagging, 35
Gallbladder, 41, 42, 59
        disorders of, 46–47
Gallbladder rupture, 47
Gallstones, 46–47
Gastric folds, 53
Gastric ulcers, 53, 55
Gastritis, 57–58
Giardia, 224–25
Gingival hyperplasia, 29–30
Gingivitis, 30–32
Glaucoma, 151, 156
Glossitis, 32
Glucagon, 98
Glucocorticoids, 100
Glucose, 98–99
Grand mal seizures, 124
Granulomas, 171–72
Grass, eating, 35
Greenstick fractures, 114
Grooming, tongue and, 23
Growth hormone, 97
Gums, 23
        gingival hyperplasia,
            29–30
        gingivitis, 30–32

Hairballs, 64
        prevention of, 57
Hair loss, 104–5
        neurodermatitis (psy-
            chogenic alopecia),
            164
Hair ring, paraphimosis due
    to, 19
Head tilt, 120
Head trauma, 119–21
Hearing process, 175–76
Heart, 85
Heart and circulatory dis-
    eases, 86–95
        aortic stenosis, 94
        atrioventricular valve
            complex malforma-
            tion, 90–91
        patent ductus arteriosus
            (PDA), 91–93
        portal caval shunt, 94–95
        vegetative endocarditis,
            88
        ventricular septal defect
            (VSD), 93–94

Heartworm, 217
Heat cycles, 2–4
Hematoma, auricular, 177–78
Hemorrhage, uterine, prolonged, 15–16
Hepatic lipidosis (fatty liver disease), 44–45
Hepatitis, 45–46
Hereditary corneal dystrophy, 150
Hereditary deafness, 183
Hernias
    diaphragmatic, 81–82
    inguinal (small intestine), 60–62
Herniated disc (slipped or ruptured disc), 116–18
Herpetic keratitis, 147–48
Himalayan cats, 141, 143, 144, 148, 157
Hookworms, 64, 65, 221–22
Hormone disorders, 97–105
Hydrocephaly, 122–23
Hydrocortisone (cortisol), 100
Hyperparathyroidism, primary, 103
Hyperthyroidism, 102–3
Hypertrophic cardiomyopathy, 86
Hypothalamus, cancer of, 100

Icterus (jaundice), 41, 45
Idiopathic miliary dermatitis, 163–64
Ileum, 59
Incubation period, defined, 227
Infant cats
    kitten mortality complex (fading kitten syndrome), 246–47
    teeth, 21, 23–25
Infections
    bladder, 190–91
    brain and spinal cord, 125–26
    conjunctivitis due to, 135
    corneal ulcers caused by, 147–48

middle ear (otitis media), 181–82
outer ear (otitis externa), 178–79
vaginal, 5
Infectious diseases, 227–47
    calicivirus, 231–32
    distemper (feline panleukopenia virus), 228–29
    fading kitten syndrome, 246–47
    feline immunodeficiency virus (feline AIDS or FIV), 241–43
    feline infectious anemia (FIA), 245–46
    feline infectious peritonitis (FIP), 235–38
    leukemia virus, feline (FeLV), 238–41
    Lyme disease (borreliosis), 234–35
    pneumonitis (parrot fever, psittacosis), 232–33
    rabies, 233–34
    rhinotracheitis virus, 229–31
    ringworm, 243–45
    terminology associated with, 227
Ingrown nails, 174
Inguinal rings and hernias, 60–61
Inhalation allergies, 168
Inherited polycystic kidneys, 188–89
Inner ear, 175
Insulin, 43, 97, 98
Intercourse, 4
Intestinal parasites, 66, 217–26
Iris, 130
    disorders of, 152–54

Jaundice (icterus), 41, 45
Jejunum, 59
Joints, 108. See also Bone and joint disorders
Juvenile cataracts, 157, 158

Keratitis, herpetic, 147–48
Kidneys, 185
    disorders of, 185–90
        acute renal disease, 186–87
        cancer, 189–90
        chronic renal disease, 187–88
        inherited polycystic kidneys, 188–89
Kidney stones, 103
Kindling, 14
Kitten mortality complex (fading kitten syndrome), 246–47
Knee joint, ruptured cruciate ligament, 115–16

Lacrimal ducts, 133
    plugged, 142–43
Lactational tetany (eclampsia), 18–19
Large intestine, 49
    anatomy of, 66
    disorders of, 66–69
        colitis, 66
        constipation, 67
        megacolon, 67–69
Laryngitis, 74–76
Larynx, 74–76
Lens, 131
    disorders of, 155–59
        cataracts, 157–58
        luxation, 156–57
        nuclear sclerosis, 158–59
Leukemia virus, feline (FeLV), 125, 238–41
Lice (pediculosis), 213–14
Lick granulomas, 171
Ligaments, 108
    cruciate (knee joint), ruptured, 115–16
Linear granuloma, 171
Lip ulcers, 171
Liver, 41
    fatty liver disease (hepatic lipidosis), 44–45
    hepatitis, 45–46
    portal caval shunt and, 94–95
    tumors, 45

Lone Star tick, 210
Lubricating glands (cerumen glands), cancer of, 167
Lung cancer, 82–83
Lungs, 79–84
Lungworms, 200, 216
Luteinizing hormone (LH), 97
Luxated patellas, 111–12
Lyme disease (borreliosis), 211, 234–35
Lymph, 197
Lymphatics, 197
Lymphatic system, 197–99
Lymph glands, 197
Lymph nodes, 197
Lymphocytes, 197
Lymphosarcoma (lymphoma), 45, 197–99

Maggots, 215–16
Magnesium, 192–94, 196
Malocclusion of teeth, 28–29
Mammary hyperplasia, 16
Mammary tumors (cancer), 9–11
Manx cats, 150
Mastitis, 16–18
Megace, 105
Megacolon, 67–69
Megaesophagus, congenital, 49–51
Megestrol acetate, 105
Meibomian gland infections, 136–37
Melanocyte-stimulating hormone (MSH), 97
Metabolism, 185
Metestrus period, 4
Metritis, acute, 9
Middle ear, 175
    infections of, 181–82
Miliary dermatitis, 163
Milk fever (eclampsia), 18–19
Mineralocorticoids, 97, 100
Mites
    ear, 179–81
    scabies, 204–6
Mitral valve, 85
Monorchidism, 20
Motion sickness, 126

Mouth
    cancer, 34
    foreign bodies in, 35–36
Mucous membranes, 71
Muscles, 107–8
Musculoskeletal system, 107–18
    bone and joint disorders, 108–15
    muscle, ligament and tendon disorders, 115–18
Myelitis, 125

Nails
    ingrown, 174
    of polydactyl cats, 111
Nasal folds, prominent, 141–42
Nasal infections, 72–73
Nervous system, 119–27
Neurodermatitis (psychogenic alopecia), 164
Nictitating membrane (third eyelid), 132, 135
    everted, 139–40
    foreign bodies behind, 140–41
Night vision, 131
Nitrogen, in urine, 186
Noradrenaline (norepinephrine), 100
Nose, 71–74
    foreign bodies in, 73–74
Nuclear sclerosis, 158–59
Nymphomania, 5
Nystagmus, 120

Odd-eyed cats, 183
Optic nerve, 131
Orchitis, 19
Osteoarthritis, 112–13
Otitis externa, 178–79
Otitis media, 181–82
Otodectes cynotis (ear mites), 208–10
Ovaban, 105
Ovarian cysts, 5–6
Ovaries, 1, 97
Ovariohysterectomy (spay), 6–9, 14, 15

Oviducts, 1
Ovulation, 4
Oxytocin, 13, 14, 16

Pancreas, 41, 43, 59, 97
    disorders of, 47–48, 98–99
Pancreatitis, 47–48
Paraphimosis, 19
Parasites, 200–226
    colon, 66
    of the heart and lungs, 216
        heartworm, 217
        lungworms, 216
    of the intestinal tract, 217–26
        coccidiosis (coccidia), 222–24
        giardia, 224–25
        hookworms, 221–22
        roundworms (ascariasis), 217–19
        tapeworms, 219–21
        toxoplasmosis, 225–26
    outer ear (ear mites), 179–81
    of the skin and ears, 200–216
        cheyletiellosis (walking dandruff), 206–8
        cuterebra fly, 215
        ear mites (otodectes cynotis), 208–10
        fleas, 200–204
        fly strike, 215–16
        lice (pediculosis), 213–14
        scabies (sarcoptic mange), 204–6
        ticks, 210–13
Parasitic enteritis, 64–65
Parathyroid gland, 103–4
Parathyroid hormone, 103
Parrot fever (psittacosis), 134
Parvovirus, 228
Patella, luxated, 111–12
Patent ductus arteriosus (PDA), 91–93

Paw, 109, 110
Pediculosis (lice), 213–14
Penis, 1, 2
    paraphimosis, 19
Peripheral nervous system
    (PNS), 119
Peritonitis
    due to bile spill, 47
    feline infectious (FIP),
        46, 235–38
Persian cats, 3, 72, 137, 141,
    144
    conjunctivitis in, 135
Persistent pupillary mem-
    brane, 153–54
Petit mal seizures, 124
Pheromones, 1
PICA (depraved appetite),
    34–35
Pink eye, 134
Pinna. See Ear flaps
Pituitary gland, 97
    cancer of, 100
Pituitary hormones, 97
Placentas, retained, 14–15
Plaque, 29, 30, 32
Plasma, 85
Platelets, 85
Pneumonia, 79
Pneumonitis, feline (parrot
    fever, psittacosis), 78,
    79–80, 232–33
Pneumothorax, 80–81
Polycystic kidneys, inherited,
    188–89
Polydactylism, 111, 174
Polyestrus, 3
Portal caval shunt, 94–95
Pregnancy, ectopic, 11–12
Proestrus, 4
Progesterones, 1, 6, 97
Prolactin hormone, 97
Prostate gland, 1, 2
Proteins, kidneys and,
    186
Psittacosis (parrot fever),
    134
Psychogenic alopecia (neu-
    rodermatitis), 164
Ptyalism (excessive drool-
    ing), 37–38
Puberty, 3

Pupil, 130–31
    persistent pupillary
        membrane, 153–54
Pyloric sphincter, 53, 56
Pyloric stenosis, 55–56
Pyometra, 5, 6–8

Rabies, 125, 233–34
Ranula (sialocele), 38–39
Rectum, 66
Red blood cells, 85
Regurgitation
    in megaesophagus, 50
    normal, 51–52
Reproductive system
    female, 1–19
        acute metritis, 9
        chronic endometri-
            tis, 8–9
        cystic endometrial
            hyperplasia, 8
        dystocia, 12–13
        eclampsia (lacta-
            tional tetany or
            milk fever), 18–19
        ectopic pregnancy,
            11–12
        heat cycles, 2–4
        mammary hyperpla-
            sia, 16
        mastitis, 16–18
        ovarian cysts, 5
        prolonged uterine
            hemorrhage, 15–16
        pyometra, 6–8
        retained placentas
            (fetal membranes),
            14–15
        uterine inertia,
            13–14
        uterine prolapse,
            14
        vaginitis, 5
    male, 1–2, 19–20
        cryptorchidism, 20
        orchitis, 19
        paraphimosis (due
            to hair ring), 19
Respiratory system, 70–84
    anatomy of, 70–71
    larynx, 74–76
    lungs, 79–84

    nose, 71–74
    trachea, 76–78
Retained placentas (fetal
    membranes), 14–15
Retina, 131
    detached, 154–55
    disorders of, 154–55
Retrobulbar abscess,
    144–45
Rhabdovirus, 233
Rhinitis, 72–73
Rhinotracheitis virus, feline,
    134, 135, 229–31
Ringworm, 243–45
Rocky Mountain Spotted
    Fever tick, 210
Rodent ulcers, 171
Roundworms (ascariasis),
    64, 65, 217–19
Ruptured cruciate ligament
    (knee joint), 115–16
Ruptured disc, 116–18

Saddle thrombi (arterial
    thromboembolism),
    88–90
Salivary glands, 21, 37
Sarcoptic mange (feline
    scabies), 204–6
Sclera, 129, 134
Seizures (epilepsy), 120,
    123–24
Sex hormones, 100
Shampoo, 163, 169, 170,
    203–4
Sialocele (ranula), 38–39
Siamese cats, 131, 148
Sight, 131–32
Sinuses, 71
Skeletal system. See Muscu-
    loskeletal system
Skin, 161
Skin disorders. See also Der-
    matitis; Parasites, of the
    skin and ears
        abscesses, 172–73
        acne, 169–70
        cancer, 166–67
        eosinophilic granuloma
            complex, 171–72
        flea hypersensitivity,
            165

frostbite, 173–74
ringworm, 243–45
Slipped disc, 116–18
Small intestine, 41
anatomy of, 59
disorders of, 59–65
foreign bodies, 62–64
parasitic enteritis,
64–65
tumors, 65
Smell, sense of, 71–72
Sneezing, 74
Sodium, 185–86
Solar dermatitis, 166
Spinal cord
infections, 125–26
tumors, 121–22
Spinose ear tick, 211
Spleen, 197
Spraying, 195
Squamous cell carcinoma,
166
Status epilepticus, 124
Sternal recumbency, 80
Steroids, 97–98, 101
Stomach
disorders of, 52–59
foreign bodies,
56–57
gastric ulcers, 53, 55
gastritis, 57–58
pyloric stenosis,
55–56
tumors, 58–59
Struvite calculi, 192–93
Stud tail (feline tail gland
hyperplasia), 162–63

Tail, stud (feline tail gland
hyperplasia), 162–63
Tapetum lucidum, 131
Tapeworms, 64, 65, 219–21
fleas and, 201
Tartar, 29, 30, 32
Taurine deficiency, 155
Tear ducts, 133
Tear glands, 133
Tears, 132, 133
plugged lacrimal ducts
and, 142
staining (epiphora),
143–44

Teeth, 21–29
abscessed roots, 26–27
cavities (caries), 25–26
fractured, 27–28
malocclusion of, 28–29
retained baby (decidu-
ous), 23–25
Testes, 97
Testicles, 1, 2
cryptorchidism, 20
orchitis, 19
Testosterone, 97
Third eyelid (nictitating
membrane), 132, 135
everted, 139–40
foreign bodies behind,
140–41
Thromboembolism, arterial
(saddle thrombi), 88–90
Thyroid gland, 97
disorders of, 102–4
Thyroid hormone, 102
Thyroid-stimulating hor-
mone (TSH), 97
Thyroxine, 97, 102
Ticks, 210–13
hard-shelled, 210–11
soft-shelled, 211
Toes, extra, 111
Tongue, 21, 23
glossitis, 32
Tonsillitis, 33
Tonsils, 33
Toxoplasmosis, 125, 225–26
Trachea, 70, 76–78
Tracheal collapse, 76–77
Tracheobronchitis, 77–78
Transmissible gastroenteritis
(TGEV), 237
Tricuspid valve, 85
Trypsin, 43
Tumors (cancer), 34
adrenal gland, 100
bone, 115
brain and spinal cord,
121–22
hypothalamus, 100
intestinal, 65
kidney, 189–90
leukemia virus, feline
(FeLV), 238–41
liver, 45

lung, 82–83
lymphosarcoma (lym-
phoma), 197–99
mammary, 9–11
mouth, 34
parathyroid glands,
104
pituitary gland, 100
skin, 166–67
small intestine, 65
stomach, 58–59
thyroid, 102–103

Ulcers
corneal, 138, 140,
146–48
gastric, 53, 55
rodent (lip), 171
Umbilical hernias, 60, 61–62
Uremia, 187
Ureter, 185, 190
Urethra, 2, 185, 190, 194–95
Urethritis, 191–92
Urinary calculi (urinary
stones or urolithiasis),
192–93
Urinary crystals, 194
Urinary system, 184–96
disorders of, 190–96.
See also Kidneys,
disorders of
feline urological
syndrome (FUS),
194–96
urethritis, 191–92
urinary calculi,
192–93
kidney and ureter dis-
orders, 185–90
Uterine contractions, 13,
14
Uterine inertia, 13–14
Uterine prolapse, 14
Uterus, 1
acute metritis, 9
chronic endometritis,
8–9
cystic endometrial
hyperplasia, 8
prolonged hemorrhage
following birth, 15–16
Uveitis, 152

Vagina, 1
Vaginal discharge, 7, 9
Vaginal flushes (douches),
  5
Vaginitis, 5
Vas deferens, 1, 2
Vegetative endocarditis,
  88
Ventricles of the heart, 85
Ventricular septal defect
  (VSD), 93–94

Vitreous fluid, 129–30,
  150–51
Vocal cords, 74
Vomiting
  foreign bodies in the
    stomach and, 56
  gastric ulcers and,
    55
  gastritis and, 58
  in pyloric stenosis, 55,
    56

regurgitation vs., 51
stomach tumors and, 58

Walking dandruff (cheyletiel-
  losis), 206–8
White blood cells, 85
Windpipe, 76. *See also* Tra-
  chea
Wood ticks, 211
Worms, 64. *See also specific
  types of worms*